SUICIDE IN PREGNANCY

George J. Kleiner, MD
Editor

Wilma Markus Greston
Associate Editor

John Wright • PSG Inc
Boston Bristol London
1984

Library of Congress Cataloging in Publication Data
Main entry under title:

Suicide in pregnancy.

Includes bibliographical references and index.
1. Pregnant women--Suicidal behavior. 2. Pregnancy, Unwanted--Psychological aspects. I. Kleiner, George J., 1926– . II. Greston, Wilma Markus. [DNLM: 1. Suicide--In pregnancy. HV 6546 S9484]
RG588.S94 1984 616.85'8445 84-3725
ISBN 0-7236-7037-4

Published simultaneously by:
John Wright • PSG Inc, 545 Great Road, Littleton, Massachusetts 01460, U.S.A.
John Wright & Sons Ltd, 823–825 Bath Road, Bristol BS4 5NU, England

Printed in United States of America

International Standard Book Number: 0-7236-7037-4

Library of Congress Catalog Card Number: 84-3725

To Edith, Jill and John,
with my loving thanks for
their help and faith

(G.J.K.)

CONTRIBUTORS

JOHN MANN ASTRACHAN, MD, FACOG
Associate Clinical Professor of Psychiatry in Obstetrics and Gynecology
The New York Hospital
Cornell Medical Center
New York, New York

NICHOLAS P. DESTOUNIS, MD, PhD, FICPM, MRC Psych, FAPM
Director, Inpatient Psychiatry
Veterans Administration Medical Center
Associate Professor of Psychiatry
Medical College of Virginia
Virginia Commonwealth University
Richmond, Virginia

IRA W. GABRIELSON, MD, MPH
Professor and Chairman
Department of Community and Preventive Medicine
Medical College of Pennsylvania
Philadelphia, Pennsylvania

JEAN M. GOODWIN, MD, MPH
Associate Professor
Department of Psychiatry
University of New Mexico School of Medicine
Albuquerque, New Mexico

WILMA MARKUS GRESTON, MT (ASCP)
Research Associate, Department of Obstetrics and Gynecology
Montefiore Medical Center
Principal Associate in Gynecology and Obstetrics
Albert Einstein College of Medicine
Bronx, New York

KERSTIN HÖÖK, MD
Professor of Psychiatry
Department of Child and Youth Psychiatry
University of Göteborg
Göteborg, Sweden

GEORGE J. KLEINER, MD, FACOG, FRCS(C)
Director, Department of Obstetrics and Gynecology
Montefiore Medical Center
North Central Bronx Hospital
Professor of Gynecology and Obstetrics
Albert Einstein College of Medicine
Bronx, New York

MAJ-BRITT ROSENBAUM, MD
Director, Human Sexuality Center
Long Island Jewish-Hillside Medical Center
New Hyde Park, New York
Associate Clinical Professor of Psychiatry
Albert Einstein College of Medicine
Bronx, New York

ALLAN J. ROSENBERG, MD
Attending Staff, Sequoia Hospital
Redwood City, California
Formerly, Clinical Associate Professor of Psychiatry
Stanford University School of Medicine
Stanford, California

BONNIE R. SAKS, MD
Assistant Professor of Psychiatry
Department of Psychiatry and Behavioral Medicine
University of South Florida College of Medicine
Tampa, Florida

HAROLD SPEERT, MD, FACOG, FACS
Assistant Attending Obstetrician and Gynecologist
Presbyterian Hospital
New York, New York

J.G. WEIR, MA, MD, FRC Psych, DPM
Consulting Psychiatrist, St. Mary's Hospital
London University
London, England

F.A. WHITLOCK, MD
Professor Emeritus of Psychiatry
University of Queensland
Brisbane, Australia

CONTENTS

ACKNOWLEDGMENTS

Appreciation is acknowledged to the following for permission to reproduce materials that appear in this volume:

American Journal of Public Health, for "Suicide Attempts in a Population Pregnant as Teen-agers," by Ira W. Gabrielson, Lorraine V. Lerman, John B. Curie, Natalie C. Tyler, James F. Jekel [1970;60(12):2289–2301].

California Medicine, now the *Western Journal of Medicine,* for "Suicide, Psychiatrists and Therapeutic Abortion," by Allan J. Rosenberg and Emmanuel Silver (1965;102:407–411).

Comprehensive Psychiatry, for "Pregnancy and Attempted Suicide," by F.A. Whitlock and J.E. Edwards [1968;9(1):1–12].

Delaware Medical Journal, for "Postpartum Psychiatric Syndromes," by Nicholas Destounis (1966;38:16–19).

The American College of Obstetricians and Gynecologists (*Obstetrics and Gynecology*) for "Severe Psychologic Disorders of the Puerperium. A Recommended Approach for the Clinical Obstetrician," by John M. Astrachan [1965;25(1):13–25].

In addition, the senior editor (G.J.K.) is particularly grateful to Dr. Joseph Hirsh who was his mentor and first collaborator on the subject. It is a pleasure to acknowledge the invaluable work of our contributors, whose efforts made this book a reality. We would like to thank Magdalene Vandiver for her assistance with the drafts of our chapters. Special thanks are owed to our longtime associate, Jennie DiLoreto, for her devotion, generosity, and skill in typing the entire manuscript.

INTRODUCTION

My curiosity about suicide and pregnancy was aroused by a clinical experience which took place about 25 years ago. A pregnant woman was admitted on our obstetrical service with a history of attempted suicide near term. She had ingested rat poison which contained phosphorus, a delayed liver toxin, as one of its ingredients, and she died before childbirth due to irreversible hepatic failure.

In the 1960s it was common to associate an unwanted pregnancy with a threat of suicide. Considering the mores at that time, and the fact that I practiced obstetrics in a busy municipal hospital in New York City, it struck me as rather odd that this should have been my first experience of a completed suicide in pregnancy. Colleagues with several lifetimes of cumulative experience in obstetrics or psychiatry, with whom I discussed this woman, failed to recall even anecdotal knowledge of suicide during pregnancy. I next looked into the health statistics of New York City with the assistance of Frieda Nelson, Assistant Director, Bureau of Health Statistics and Analysis (New York City Department of Health), and that, too, failed to reveal anything of significance, as I found only one recorded instance of suicide in pregnancy in this large urban population during the preceding five years.

Standard textbooks of obstetrics and psychiatry did not recognize the existence of suicide in pregnancy in any meaningful fashion. It seemed timely to review the subject then, as in the late 1960s, attempts were being made to liberalize abortion laws in the United States. The danger of suicide as a result of an unwanted pregnancy was one of the many cogent arguments in the debate. I kept a modest interest in the subject throughout the years, and from time to time presented update reviews on suicide during pregnancy at a variety of international conferences and university lectures.* It became apparent to me that there was enough peripheral curiosity regarding suicide in pregnancy to sustain continued involvement.

*London, England—Fifth International Conference for Suicide Prevention, September 24–27, 1969; Chicago, Illinois—Special Presentation at the 1979 Annual Meeting of the American Psychiatric Association, May 14–18, 1979; Oxford, England—Nuffield Department of Obstetrics and Gynaecology, University of Oxford, August 18, 1980; Berlin, West Germany—Sixth International Congress of Psychosomatic Obstetrics and Gynecology, September 2–6, 1980; Toronto, Canada—Fourth Tri-District Annual Meeting of the American College of Obstetricians and Gynecologists, September 23–27, 1980.

As my coeditor and I delved deeper, we became increasingly aware of how little information was available. Most of what was published surfaced only as part of the discussion of suicide in general. Obstetrical awareness and input was almost totally lacking, as an occasional incident of a suicide in association with pregnancy specifically did not warrant or stimulate sufficient curiosity. Quite understandably, suicide in pregnancy remained the purview of the psychiatrist and most information which could be culled out was obtained from their literature. A prodigious amount of published material on suicide in general was found in textbooks, psychiatrically oriented journals, and sociological/statistical literature. What was missing was a text, with a comprehensive list of references, specifically oriented toward suicide in association with pregnancy, so as to bring into a single publication whatever pertinent information on the subject was available. This book aims to be of assistance to obstetricians, psychiatrists, social workers, and sociologists as an aid in clinical assessment as well as in education. It may facilitate a convenient overview of the subject in the event that a clinical situation of attempted or completed suicide should occur in association with pregnancy. We were, therefore, enormously pleased to be given the opportunity by John Wright • PSG Inc. to bring the subject of suicide during pregnancy into a meaningful whole.

We have attempted to review suicide in pregnancy from the demographic as well as the psychiatric point of view. Not infrequently, common themes weave in and out of the fabric of the presentations by individual contributors. Special effort was made, however, to identify each author with his or her special expertise on a specific topic or group of subjects. The goal was to gather pertinent information from those authors currently recognized for their interest in suicide during pregnancy. With one or two exceptions, these were mostly psychiatrists, many with national and international reputations and distinguished academic careers. When appropriate, published articles have been reprinted when no fresh data were available and we thought that this information was still relevant.

Even though suicide during pregnancy may be a rare phenomenon, the problem is of significance because of its broader relationship to the issues of unwanted pregnancy and abortion. Before liberalization of abortion laws, it often had been proposed that unwanted pregnancy could lead to suicide. Much of the data on completed and attempted suicide in association with pregnancy date back to those times when abortions were done either illegally, strictly for maternal health reasons, or as approved by special hospital boards on psychiatric grounds—times when illegal abortion could have been considered tantamount to attempted suicide because of the high risk of medical complication. The literature and the dialogue reflect past and current conflicts and confusions.

The debate revolves around a variety of legal and psychiatric opinions concerning the potential of suicide either due to unwanted pregnancy or because of preexisting psychiatric conditions. This material once more becomes timely because of current pressures in the United States to revert back to more restrictive practices regarding elective interruption of pregnancy.

The association of potential suicide and teen-age pregnancy also warrants special attention. In the United States, the problem of children bearing children assumed epidemic proportions. The article of Gabrielson points to the dangers of subsequent suicide in those women who had children as teen-agers. Although tangential to the discussion of suicide during pregnancy, this paper demonstrates the significantly higher risk of future suicides for these women. It appears that among the long-term sequelae of attempted suicide in pregnancy are congenital abnormalities, psychologic deprivation, and child abuse which may even lead to infanticide. The impression exists that it is the younger woman who is more likely to attempt and also to succeed in committing suicide. In fact, there are a few recent case reports in which the women who killed themselves while pregnant were under 18, and one was as young as 14.

Our intuitive belief is that attempted suicide in pregnancy is underreported and needs to be appropriately studied in a prospective manner. Studies of completed suicide during pregnancy could be improved by some standardization of data collection, with uniformity of reporting statistical information. To get a true measure of the potential for suicide during pregnancy, it would be particularly valuable to obtain a postmortem examination on every woman of childbearing age whose death appears, in any way, to be self-inflicted. Like others, we believe that completed suicide in pregnancy is a rare event. It is likely that it will remain a medical curiosity for the foreseeable future.

SECTION I

HISTORICAL AND LITERARY PERSPECTIVES

This section reflects attempts to review suicide associated with pregnancy from the vantage of history and classic Western literature. According to Dr. Speert, an authority on the history of obstetrics and gynecology, and other distinguished scholars in the field of history of medicine, no significant work on this subject can be found, although much has been written on birth control, abortion, and childbirth in general as far back as the Bible.

Despite the myriad novels and plays over the past two centuries, with few exceptions, there is surprising lack of literary allusion to suicide in pregnancy. This void is particularly difficult to understand when one considers that sex and the often resultant unwanted pregnancy are problems inherent in our social condition. Since commonly accepted folklore considered that suicide is used as a solution to the problem of unwanted pregnancy, one might have expected that it would have been dealt with more frequently in literature. There are examples of suicides of young women who might have been pregnant, but the suicide is not attributed to pregnancy per se, eg, Ophelia, Lucretia. In recent writings there are suggestions, perhaps influenced by women's rights movements, that having an abortion in the days when it was illegal was tantamount to attempting suicide. For example, in the novel, The Company of Women, *Mary Gordon (1980) explicitly makes the point that going for an illegal abortion is a suicidal act. There are other sporadic descriptions which concerned real events and, by virtue of the principles involved, became "causes celebres" of the time. Dr. Goodwin, a psychiatrist who is one of the few current authorities on suicide during pregnancy in the United States, elaborates on some of these in this section. In addition, using these literary allusions as background, Dr. Goodwin further elaborates on the timing and methods of suicide during pregnancy in contemporary cases of suicide in New Mexico in Chapter 8.*

CHAPTER 1

SUICIDE IN PREGNANCY AND MORTUARY CUSTOMS IN HISTORY AND LITERATURE

HAROLD SPEERT

Early in the 6th century BC, it is told, there lived in Rome the fair Lucretia, wife of Lucius Collatinus, renowned for her beauty and conjugal fidelity. Unable to resist his primal urge, Sextus Tarquinius, son of a neighboring noble ravished her; whereupon Lucretia summoned her father and her husband. "They came . . . ," Shakespeare wrote in his "Argument" affixed to the original edition (1594) of his poem *The Rape of Lucrece* (Shakespeare, 1821), "and finding the outraged heroine attired in mourning habit, demanded the cause of her sorrow. She first taking an oath of them for her revenge, revealed the actor, and the whole manner of his dealing . . ."

Believing herself pregnant, Lucretia lamented:

"The remedy indeed to do me good,
Is to let forth my foul, defiled blood.
Poor hand, why quiver'st thou at this decree?
Honour thyself to rid me of this shame;
For if I die, my honour lives in thee,
But if I live, thou liv'st in my defame;
Since thou could'st not defend thy loyal dame,
And wast afear'd to scratch her wicked foe,
Kill both thyself and her for yielding so.
This said, from her be-tumbled couch she starteth,
To find some desperate instrument of death:
But this no slaughter-house no tool imparteth,
To make more vent for passage of her breath;
Which, thronging through her lips, so vanisheth
As smoke from Aetna, that in air consumes,
Or that which from discharged cannon fumes.
In vain, quoth she, I live and seek in vain
Some happy mean to end a hapless life.
I fear'd by Tarquin's falchion to be slain,
Yet for the self-same purpose seek a knife:
But when I fear'd, I was a loyal wife;

So am I now: — O no, that cannot be;
Of that true type hath Tarquin rifled me.
O! that is gone for which I sought to live,
And therefore now I need not fear to die.
To clear this spot by death, at least I give
A badge of fame to slander's livery;
A dying life to living infamy:
Poor helpless help, the treasure stol'n away,
To burn the guiltless casket where it lay!
Well, well, dear Collatine, thou shalt not know
The stained taste of violated troth;
I will not wrong thy true affection so,
To flatter thee with an infringed oath;
This bastard graff shall never come to growth:
He shall not boast, who did thy stock pollute,
That thou art doting father of his fruit.
Nor shall he smile at thee in secret thought,
Nor laugh with his companions at thy state;
But thou shalt know thy interest was not bought
Basely with gold, but stolen from forth thy gate.
For me, I am the mistress of my fate;
And with my trespass never will dispense,
Till life to death acquit my forc'd offence.

* * * * * * *

My honour I'll bequeath unto the knife
That wounds my body so dishonoured.
'Tis honour to deprive dishonour'd life;
The one will live, the other being dead:
So of shame's ashes shall my fame be bred;
For in my death I murder shameful scorn:
My shame so dead, mine honour is new-born.
Dear lord of that dear jewel I have lost,
What legacy shall I bequeath to thee?
My resolution, love, shall be thy boast,
By whose example thou reveng'd may'st be.
How Tarquin must be us'd, read it in me:
Myself, thy friend, will kill myself, thy foe,
And, for my sake, serve thy false Tarquin so.
This brief abridgment of my will I make:
My soul and body to the skies and ground;
My resolution, husband, do thou take;
Mine honour be the knife's, that makes my wound;
My shame be his that did my fame confound;
And all my fame that lives, disbursed be
To those that live, and think no shame of me.

* * * * * * *

Besides, the life and feeling of her passion
She hoards, to spend when he is by to hear her;
When sighs and groans and tears may grace the fashion
Of her disgrace, the better so to clear her
From that suspicion which the world might bear her.
    To shun this blot, she would not blot the letter
    With words, till action might become them better.

* * * * * * *

Here with a sigh, as if her heart would break,
She throws forth Tarquin's name: *He, he,* she says,
But more than *he* her poor tongue could not speak;
Till after many accents and delays,
Untimely breathings, sick and short assays,
    She utters this: He, he, fair lords, 'tis he,
    That guides this hand to give this wound to me.
Even here she sheathed in her harmless breast
A harmful knife, that thence her soul unsheath'd:
That blow did bail it from the deep unrest
Of that polluted prison where it breath'd:
Her contrite sighs unto the clouds bequeath'd
    Her winged sprite, and through her wounds doth fly
    Life's lasting date from cancel'd destiny.
Stone-still, astonish'd with this deadly deed.
Stood Collatine and all his lordly crew;
Till Lucrece' father that beholds her bleed,
Himself on her self-slaughter'd body threw;
And from the purple fountain Brutus drew
    The murderous knife, and as it left the place,
    Her blood, in poor revenge, held it in chase;
And bubbling from her breast, it doth divide
In two slow rivers, that the crimson blood
Circles her body in on every side,
Who like a late-sack'd island vastly stood,
Bare and unpeopled, in this fearful flood.
    Some of her blood still pure and red remain'd,
    And some look'd black, and that false Tarquin stain'd."

The legend of Lucretia, in varying detail, had been related by Livy (59 BC–17 AD), Ovid (43 BC–17 AD), Chaucer (1340?–1400) and others. A *ballet* called *"The Grievous Complaint of Lucrece"* was licensed to John Alde in 1558, "A Ballad of the Death of Lucryssia" to James Roberts in 1569, and another ballad of the same tale was printed in 1576. These accounts, which doubtless provided the basis for Shakespeare's poem, portray a rare example of suicide in pregnancy. Sixteenth-century woodcuts depicting Lucretia's death appeared in Schäferlin's *Livius* (Figure 1-1) and Sebastian Munster's *Cosmographei.*

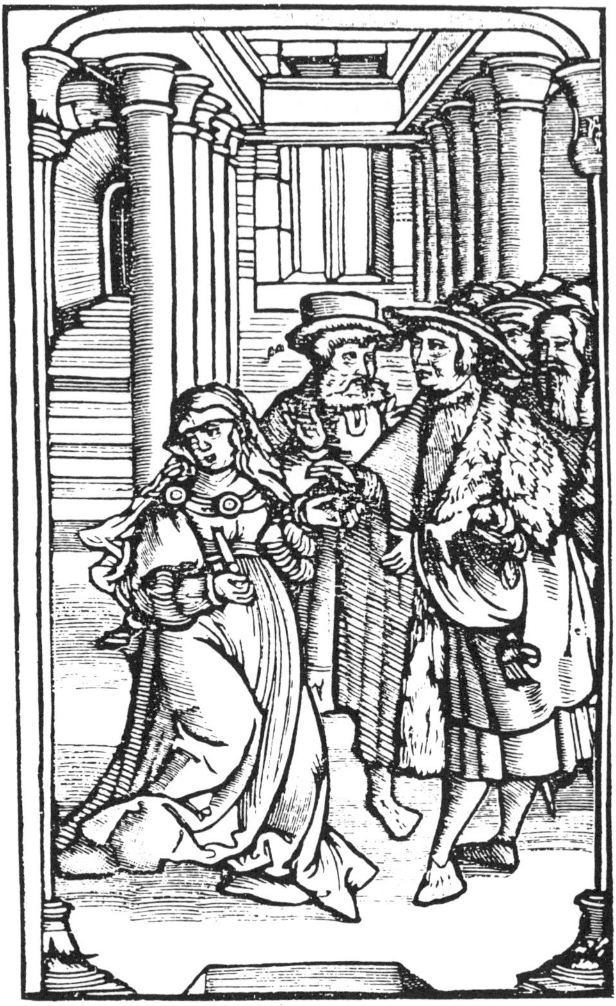

Figure 1-1 The suicide of Lucretia, 16th century woodcut (Ploss, 1905).

The monumental historic and anthropologic study of woman by Ploss and Bartels (1905), containing a chapter of 57 pages on "Woman in Death," with eight pages devoted to suicide, makes no mention of suicide in pregnancy. Most common causes of self-inflicted death among women have been unrequited or lost love and the threat of violation of virginity. Suicide was judged to be less frequent among women of primitive cultures than in so-called civilized societies.

American Indian women disappointed in love jumped to their death from cliffs. Bereaved squaws among the Tautin Indians of Oregon sought in suicide an escape from the humiliation of widowhood. Until the middle of the 19th century, women of the Wahpeton and Sisseton tribes, members of the eastern division of the Sioux (Dakota) Indians, commonly hanged themselves from a tree after the death of a favorite child (Yarrow, 1881). Other social and ritualistic reasons for suicide among American Indian women included forced marriage, maltreatment by husband, and childlessness.

In mid-19th-century China women often took their lives after the death of a husband, either because of emotional attachment to the departed, poverty, or fear of maltreatment by the dead husband's relatives (Doolittle, 1868). Some took a large dose of opium or other poison, then lay down beside their deceased spouse. Others starved, drowned, or hanged themselves in public. Public suicide by a widow was considered honorable and usually attracted a crowd of spectators. Incense and candles were burned in the temple on the first and fifteenth of each Chinese month in honor of bereaved betrothed women who had hanged themselves to avoid another engagement or an unmarried future.

During the reign of Emperor Taukwang, Katscher (1881) told, 15 or more young girls, upon learning that they have been betrothed by their parents, drowned themselves in a tributary of the Canton River and were buried together in what came to be known as "the Virgins' Grave." In a neighboring village in 1873, eight other girls, after dressing in their finest clothes and binding themselves together, committed mass suicide in similar fashion.

An article in a Tientsin newspaper of January 3, 1888, related the pledge of a group of unmarried girls in the province of Kwangtung, members of the Golden Orchids Society, vowing not to permit sexual intercourse with their future husbands until every member of the group was married. In the face of force the virginal members of the society resorted to suicide, always in groups of seven. On one occasion, seven girls poised themselves on the bank of a river at midnight, to perish in the current, but at the critical moment one withdrew, to save herself. As a result, it was stated, six mourning ghosts continued to haunt the water's edge, deploring the action of their unfaithful sister.

CHAPTER 2

THE MEANING AND THE MADNESS IN THE METHOD OF SUICIDE IN PREGNANCY: Literary Allusions

JEAN GOODWIN

In the play *Hamlet* (Shakespeare, 1957), Polonius says of the young prince, "Though this be madness, yet there is method in it" (Act II, Scene II). One often has a similar feeling about the suicides that occur during pregnancy. Such suicides initially strike observers as irrationally against nature, and yet after careful study of a particular case, one begins to see a difficult-to-define symmetry in the action.

The play *Hamlet* is an appropriate starting point for an exploration of the meanings of suicide in pregnancy and of the clues to those meanings to be found in the suicidal method. *Hamlet* has at times been performed with an Ophelia dressed to appear obviously pregnant. This reading of the play makes sense of Ophelia's persistent pursuit of Hamlet, despite his disinterest, and of her father Polonius's involvement in that pursuit. It sheds a different light on the constant and explicit sexual references in conversations between Hamlet and Ophelia and lends method to Ophelia's despair and madness when Hamlet's murder of her father and Hamlet's own exile destroy any possibility of a timely marriage. If one seeks for method in Ophelia's mad scene (Act IV, Scene V), one finds her talking of loss of virginity, of false promises of marriage, and of fear about the future. ("We know what we are, but know not what we may be." "I hope all will be well. We must be patient.") In the Queen's description of Ophelia's death by drowning (Act IV, Scene VIII), Ophelia is described as playing with her flowers and singing while her sodden clothes pull her down into the water. Ophelia has turned her back so resolutely on fears about her future that she is oblivious to danger and can readily enter that death about which Hamlet himself has been so ambivalent. Shakespeare has created a kingdom of Denmark which is so corrupt and which faces the future in such disarray that a pregnant Ophelia is even less likely than a virginal Ophelia to find support either from Hamlet or from his parents. The royal guards fail to rescue her as she is drowning, perhaps because Hamlet's heir would have been an embarrassment.

Literature and history are difficult but enticing sources of information about suicide in pregnancy (Slochower, 1975; Feggetter, 1980). Fiction offers us characters born out of the symbolizing craft of their authors as well as from contemporary beliefs about human behavior. Thus fiction offers a statistical surfeit of female suicides and of completed (as opposed to attempted) suicides because such suicides are dramatically successful (Feggetter, 1980). However, certain literary suicides, such as the suicide of Cio Cio San in Puccini's *Madame Butterfly* (Feggetter, 1980) or Werther's suicide in Goethe's *The Sorrows of Young Werther* (Slochower, 1975) illuminate with empathic detail important culture-bound clinical syndromes of suicide.

In studying suicide in pregnancy, one must look to history and literature for much of this empathic detail. With even greater frequency than in other types of suicide, suicides in pregnancy are concealed (or the pregnancy is concealed or denied), notes are not left, and the victim has not shared her plight or her decision to end it by suicide with a physician or with a family member (Goodwin and Harris, 1979). The bare facts of the method used and the time, place, and witnesses of the death are often the only indications of the underground turmoil that produced the suicide.

Before examining such raw data from contemporary suicides (Chapter 8), we will review three additional cases in which writers and biographers have added, to the bare bones of method and circumstances, some direct and symbolic information about motivation.

METHODS OF SUICIDE IN PREGNANCY IN THREE FAMOUS LITERARY AND HISTORICAL CASES

These three literary cases are presented in the format that will be used later for contemporary cases of suicide in pregnancy. In reviewing these cases, an attempt will be made to dissect similarities, differences, and motivational sequences which can help us to make sense of the more skeletal information available in contemporary cases.

Case A

Maeve O'Riorden (Spring, 1938) was a 25-year-old Irish-born actress and London music hall entertainer. In the autumn of 1916 she revived a friendship with a childhood sweetheart, Oliver Essex, after he was decorated for bravery in the Battle of the Somme. Part of her motivation was a sense of responsibility to any young soldier soon to face danger and possibly death; another part was a desire to distract Oliver from his previous lover, a woman he had "taken away" from his novelist father, William Essex, the man to whom Maeve was most closely attached. Maeve believed William could resume his former romance if Oliver were distracted; this, however, did not occur. In January 1917, on the night Oliver was to return to the trenches, Maeve lost her virginity to him. A week later he was taken prisoner by the Germans. By late February she realized that she was pregnant. Oliver's father offered to care for her and the child and suggested he marry her. She rejected this, fearing she would become once again a pawn in the jealous triangles that this father and son engineered. She asked Oliver's father to see her in what turned out to be her last performance for her beloved troops. She was anxious lest the pregnancy dull her performance. Later that night she took an overdose of sleeping pills. Mr. Essex and a physician friend concealed both the suicide and the pregnancy, letting it be known that she had died of "heart trouble" exacerbated by fatigue caused by her devotion to the troops. Maeve's patriotic devotion to the British war effort was at odds with the Irish patriotism of the O'Riorden family, some of whom were actively fighting for Irish independence.

Case B

Hedda Gabler Tesman (McFarland, 1966) was the 29-year-old wife of a medieval scholar, Dr. Jorgen Tesman. She married Tesman in the 1890s after her father, General Gabler, was disgraced by scandal and died penniless. She felt forced into the marriage by her financial plight, and a six-month wedding trip convinced her that she would be utterly bored by her husband. On their return home, she felt left out of the Tesman family circle which included Jorgen, his two aunts (one of whom was dying), and the family servant. Hedda gravitated to the worldly Judge Brack, an old friend of her father's, and to a former suitor, Ejlert Lovborg, another historian who was in competition with Tesman for a professorship. When Tesman told Hedda that they would have to economize because of the chance that Lovborg, not Tesman, would win the professorship, Hedda said that she could amuse herself cheaply with her father's dueling pistols. She threatened Judge Brack with these pistols and had previously threatened to shoot Lovborg when he was courting her. Hedda repeatedly rebuffed hints from the old aunts and from the judge that she discuss her now obvious pregnancy. Tesman, characteristically, failed to notice the pregnancy. Hedda felt trapped in her marriage and tried to enter vicariously into the unconventional life-style that Lovborg had established with his woman friend Thea. It was as though Hedda felt she could possess that more interesting life by controlling Lovborg. Hedda tried to disrupt Lovborg's friendship with Thea, to tempt him back into alcoholism, and, finally, by burning Lovborg's book manuscript and, giving him one of her pistols, she tried to tempt him to suicide.

She lied to Tesman, saying she did these things because her pregnancy had driven her to extreme loyalty to her husband. Lovborg's suicide was not the aesthetic triumph for which Hedda hoped; he shot himself in the abdomen in a brothel. Judge Brack recognized the death weapon as Hedda's pistol and threatened to link her to the scandal unless she became his mistress. Tesman moved even farther from Hedda as he joined Thea in recreating Lovborg's manuscript. While Brack, Tesman, and Thea were in the house, Hedda went into another room and shot herself in the head with the remaining dueling pistol.

Case C

Jeanne Hebuterne (Sichel, 1967) was a 22-year-old Parisian former art student, eight months pregnant with her second child by her alcoholic, artist lover Amedeo Modigliani. Their first child, 14 months old, had been placed with a wet nurse since age 3 months. Jeanne presented at a maternity clinic for hospitalization on January 24, 1920, a few hours after her lover died of tuberculous meningitis. She was told that "her time had not yet come."

For the week prior to his death, Modigliani had been delirious; Jeanne had lain beside him in their cold attic, sharing meals of sardines and wine with him on their mattress. She had made sketches of herself committing suicide either by knifing herself in the breast or by leaping. She had told one friend that her lover wanted her to join him in death so that he could paint more portraits of her. Another friend had seen a knife under her pillow. She had visited the hospital to see his body and had been felt to be "too calm."

After being refused hospitalization at the maternity clinic, Jeanne was taken by her father to the Hebuterne family home. Jeanne's Catholic bourgeois parents had never approved of her affair and spoke bitterly about the Jewish Modigliani. They had not been mollified when Modigliani signed a statement that Jeanne was his common-law wife. It is not clear what happened that night. Some speculate that the Hebuternes forbade Jeanne to attend Modigliani's funeral or that they ordered her to leave home forever on the next day. Others say that her artist brother foiled at least one suicide attempt. At 4 AM on the day after her lover's death, Jeanne jumped from a fifth-story window of her family home and died instantly. Friends said that she must have floated down from the window like an angel in her white nightgown. One measure of the family split was that, when a workman brought her body to the door, he was not allowed to bring it inside. Ten years after her death, the parents finally agreed to rebury Jeanne next to her lover, Modigliani.

What questions arise from a study of these detailed literary and historical case histories? The methods are dramatic, in two cases violent, and are intricately bound to the network of motivations for the suicide. The three suicides have been arranged with the one occurring earliest in pregnancy first. The suicide early in pregnancy was the only one which involved a nonviolent method. All three women had been in one way or another (imprisonment, alienation, death) deserted by the father of the child, and all were estranged from their parents (by political disagreement, death, or family conflict). All three had paternal supports available; Maeve could have married her child's grandfather; Tesman and his family were ready to smother Hedda Gabler with affection; and it is likely that Jeanne would have been accepted by Modigliani's family. Yet, for various reasons, these supports were unacceptable. All would be separated, by having the child, from a valued world that they had sacrificed to create; Maeve would lose her role as every soldier's favorite sweetheart; Hedda could no longer be the envied belle who manipulated men; Jeanne would have to face the loss of her life with Modigliani. Each of these women was surrounded by death: Maeve by the soldiers' dying in World War I and in the Irish Rebellion; Hedda by the deaths of her father, of Lovborg, of her husband's aunt; and Jeanne by her lover's progressive and fatal illness. It is as if each one chose to join the dead with whom they were familiar rather than await the unknown fetus in an environment which was no longer supportive.

It may be significant that all of these suicides in pregnancy took place prior to 1921, or this may simply represent sampling error due to the author's literary tastes. It does seem that, although this fluctuates, the absolute level of societal support for the pregnant woman has increased since 1787, when one of the first American suicides in pregnancy was reported (Jones, 1980). A Mrs. Tyler in Massachusetts, a widow several months pregnant, took rat poison and died, a week after a fellow woman citizen was sentenced to death by hanging for the infanticide of a bastard child. The decriminalization of bastardy and, more recently, the legalization of abortion and the provision of financial support to single mothers would seem to reduce some of the external stress on these already internally stressed pregnant women.

SECTION II

DEMOGRAPHIC, CULTURAL, AND SOCIAL FACTORS

Even though completed suicide during pregnancy has been exceedingly rare throughout the world in modern times, better insight into the phenomenon may be gained by examination of the many intertwined elements which may influence a pregnant woman to commit suicide. The chapter on cultural, religious, and ethnic influences is devoted to reviewing these factors.

In the chapter on demographic and statistical factors, we reviewed the difficulties in gathering statistics on suicide in pregnancy as a reflection of similar problems encountered when collecting data on suicide in general. What data were available from surveys and individual case reports, mostly from the United States and Europe, were compiled in an effort to give a broad overview of the subject. At the start of the book, we had had high hopes of obtaining some hard data about the frequency and complexity of suicide in the Far East. There were hints that suicide, including suicide among pregnant women, is particularly frequent in Japan and China. We failed to obtain any supportive information through a thorough search of the literature, correspondence with scholars in the field, and personal emissaries to Japan. There is some new evidence that women who trace their origins to the Indian subcontinent, but reside in such far-distant places as England, Kenya, South Africa, or the Fiji Islands, are particularly prone to suicide in pregnancy. For future researchers, the cultural, ethnic, and even religious differences could form the basis for a more definitive study of this deviant, but rare, behavior in the pregnant female.

Dr. Weir's contribution is the largest and most comprehensive report on suicide during pregnancy available in all literature on the subject. In his chapter, Dr. Weir uses case histories to illustrate some common denominators in the different subgroups of patients. He also discusses the issue of designation of suicide versus accidental death which must play havoc in statistical reporting in many societies. We use his data in our chapter on demographic and statistical factors, where they add significantly to the variety of compiled statistics.

Dr. Weir's chapter reflects his interest and shows the care with which such statistical analyses are gathered in England and Wales. The coroners' reports and the routine performance of a detailed autopsy in cases of suicide or accidental death allowed for unique analysis of case histories of a relatively large number of women who committed suicide during pregnancy in London. The availability of such reports demonstrates a national commitment to gathering statistics in a detailed manner. In fact, the Reports on Confidential Enquiries into Maternal Deaths in England and Wales, triennial reports of the coroners' data which have been published since 1952, are unique among national statistics in identifying suicide during pregnancy as a separate entity.

Dr. Whitlock's chapter reflects his lifelong commitment to the study of suicide and attempted suicide. He is recognized as one of the leading authorities on suicide during pregnancy in the world. His earlier work is among the most frequently quoted reports in the literature. In his chapter he focuses on interpersonal relationships, marital status, and preexisting mental disease which may be possible provoking factors of suicide in association with pregnancy.

CHAPTER 3

CULTURAL, RELIGIOUS, AND ETHNIC INFLUENCES

GEORGE J. KLEINER
WILMA MARKUS GRESTON

There is no body of literature that focuses on ethnic, religious, and cultural factors specifically in association with suicide during pregnancy. In reviewing the world literature on suicide in general, it appears that there are differences in certain groups which, in like fashion, may influence the predisposition to suicide in the pregnant female. In some instances, social pressures appear to be of importance.

Many of the articles on suicide did not identify pregnancy specifically, although mention of attempted or completed suicide during pregnancy is made occasionally. The role that pregnancy might play on the causation of suicide can only be considered against the broader background of a given society; while historical, ethnic, religious, moral, social, and political factors must enter into such consideration, there are insufficient data to draw any meaningful conclusions.

In modern times, completed suicide during pregnancy has been exceedingly rare throughout the world. This review is presented in an effort to understand influences on women across a variety of cultures and geographic areas throughout the world which might predispose the pregnant woman to commit suicide.

PRIMITIVE SOCIETIES

There are almost no available statistics on suicide during pregnancy in primitive societies, although the subject of suicide in these people is well discussed (Dublin, 1963; Giddens, 1971). In *The Sociology of Suicides, a Selection of Readings*, edited by Anthony Giddens (1971), there is no reference to suicide during pregnancy in primitive societies. On the contrary, it appears that primitive societies place a premium on the value of childbearing. Indeed, they consider pregnancy as being proof of a man's virility, and it underlies the actual value or importance of a family. For instance, in the article, *Suicide Among the Gisu*, La Fontaine (1971) reports that in this African society the woman's position depends on the fulfillment of her role as a mother. While she is still capable of bearing children, a woman is of value to the community. Firth (1971) alludes to possible suicide during pregnancy in Tikopia society, an isolated, primitive Polynesian community in the western Pacific, when young women are shamed by pregnancy in which the male lover will either not acknowledge his responsibility or will not marry his mistress.

In the article, *Psychiatric Disorders Among Aborigines of the Australian Western Desert*, Jones and Horne (1973) surveyed 959 Aborigine men, women, and children of four isolated missions. Most Australian Aborigines now live in semipermanent camps around missions, having abandoned their nomadic existence, but the survey gives insight into their psychiatric disorders when they were nomadic. This group contains some of the most primitive people to be found in modern Australia, ie, those least affected by Western influences. The prevalence of psychiatric illness is lower than in Western communities. The authors point out specifically that no cases of suicide were found among these very primitive people, although one case of puerperal psychosis is listed.

URBAN AND RURAL AFRICA

Suicide in Africa has been relatively uncommon. Kiev (1979), in a broad view of transcultural perspectives of suicide in general, suggests that the advent of technology and modernization has led to increased rates, especially among the educated and professional classes. He points out that the dramatic changes in life-style from rural/tribal to urban have disrupted religious traditions and tribal brotherhoods and created much stress. Even so, the frequency of suicide among Africans under Western and urban influences is still very much less than in European societies.

Gelfand (1976) comes to a similar conclusion in his study of *Suicide and Attempted Suicide in the Urban and Rural African in Rhodesia*, in terms of ethnic and cultural characteristics, ie, that suicide remains more common in the European than in the African in Rhodesia. Similar to the Europeans, attempted suicide was significantly more frequent among the girls. Yet, in the three years of the study, the author reported no instance of suicide during pregnancy.

In the indigenous African population, Gelfand (1976) showed that suicide is more frequent among the rural population than among townspeople. This is in contrast to Kiev (1979), who states that there is evidence that social breakdown, which appears mainly in crowded areas and shantytowns of Africa, could lead to increased incidence in this group. However, both agree that the traditional or rural African population is relatively free of either suicide or attempted suicide.

FAR EAST ASIA

Price and Karim (1975) reviewed suicide in Fiji in a two-year period in the early 1970s. The data showed a much higher incidence of suicide in Fiji Indians (immigrants from the Indian subcontinent) than in other races, especially Melanesians (Polynesian in origin). The incidence in Fiji Indian females was particularly high, especially in the 15- to 24-year-old age group; two were pregnant. In the Fiji Indian population, a positive correlation between suicide and rural residence and a negative correlation between suicide and Moslem religion was found. The ratio of Indian to other races was 41:1 and, among these, the religious difference, Hindu to Moslem, was 5:1. Sharp racial, ethnic, and religious differences can influence the incidence of suicide within a small geographic area populated by a variety of races and religions. Although Price and Karim (1975) concluded that there is a racial difference which would account for the incidence of suicide, it might be that the cultural and social characteristics of the population of Fiji are of importance also.

Chi-Pang Wen (1974) wrote on the secular suicidal trend in postwar Japan and Taiwan, in particular, about high female suicidal deaths. He considers it to be a health problem of epidemic proportions. In discussing women in Japan and Taiwan, he stresses that

> in general (they) face the following difficulties in an exaggerated way—the social intolerance toward divorce, the bleak prospect of remarriage for a woman, the highly held value of chastity, the lack of sex education, the 'official' taboo on sexual freedom coexisting with rampant sexual promiscuity, the culturally male-dominant chauvinistic attitude, and the wide economic status differentials aggravating the sex differentials.

He feels that sex plays a significant role in suicidal etiology, yet he does not mention suicide during pregnancy. In the same report, he discussed suicide rates in young Chinese and Japanese residing in Hawaii. Rates of suicide were much lower among those of similar ethnic background in Hawaii than in like groups residing in Japan and Taiwan. In general, they were comparable to rates of suicides of the Hawaiian whites. Yet, despite a well-annotated and well-supported statistical analysis on a significant number of suicides over a 15-year period, again he does not allude to a single case of suicide in pregnancy.

Iga et al (1975) discussed why "young Japanese females had the highest suicide rate in the world until the end of the 1960s, and it is still extremely high." This "extraordinarily high suicide rate for Japanese females was explained in terms of the vulnerability of their personality, social conditions, and role conflict." The vulnerability was related "to socialization that emphasizes dependence, the domestic role of women, and negative views of life and social resources." The latter was assumed because of the fatalistic teaching of Buddhism. They write:

> The social conditions significant in their suicides were poverty and outcaste status; failure in performing the domestic and schoolwork roles; and rejection by parent or husband. The role conflict of young Japanese females was considered on three levels: (a) personality traits in conflict with the traditional conception of femininity; (b) the historical conflict between merchant and samurai cultures; and (c) the conflict produced by rapid modernization.

Again, there is no identification of suicide during pregnancy.

In a comparative study of completed suicide in the United States and in Japan, Joseph Hirsh (Kleiner and Hirsh, 1969), an earlier collaborator and mentor, found some striking differences in the suicide pattern in the two cultures. He points out in his *Cultural Determinants of Suicide: The Perspective of the Japanese* that the rate for female suicides of all ages is the highest in the world (Hirsh, 1966). In his review of medical examiners' data in the United States, he, like others, found a virtual absence of suicide among pregnant women. In Japan, however, suicide in pregnant women was a common event and not the exception (Kleiner and Hirsh, 1969).

"Shinju" or double suicide (for example, mother and infant or husband and wife) was apparently also common. It should be considered that there may be a possible relationship between suicide in pregnant women (with fetus in utero) and shinju, as this concept of common suicides of loved ones is accepted in Japan (J. Hirsh, personal communication, July 1969). Double suicide may be a part of a greater tendency of the Japanese to use suicide as a solution to personal problems (Hirsh, 1966). In addition, the concept of saving face is often a central feature of suicide in the Far East (Hirsh, 1960).

In Japan, until recently, suicide was not only an acceptable social behavior, firmly integrated in the national religion, but encouraged under certain circumstances. Harakiri or "belly-cutting," which is also known as bushido in the Shintu religion, is a Japanese form of suicide and part of their code of honor. According to Ilsa Veith (1969), "not every Japanese suicide is harakiri. In fact, it is a very rare form of suicide and belongs to the feudal past; it was practiced among the samurai in connection with their concept of honor." Nevertheless, until recently, the suicide rate in Japanese women between the ages of 15 and 24 was about 18 times higher than for the same ages in the United States (Wen, 1974) and was the highest among all nations in modern times.

In an effort to review current trends, repeated attempts were made to obtain statistical data through personal emissaries and communication with Japanese scholars. Unfortunately, they were unsuccessful, and we have no recent information as to what extent pregnancy takes part in this phenomenal incidence of suicide in the Far East.

In modern China, there are other serious stresses facing young people, in particular, women of childbearing age. The stringent birth-control policy of limiting new families to a single child versus the desirability to produce male children may, in fact, lead to suicide. In an August 1, 1982, *New York Times* article, "Old Nemesis Haunts China on Birth Plan," dateline Peking, Christopher Wren (1982) describes the ordeal of women who give birth to a daughter. Because of the country's stringent family-planning program, Chinese families press more than ever for a son. This apparently leads to abandonment and even infanticide in the case of female babies. It is the mistreatment of the mothers which seems to get more attention, however. Wren (1982) describes a recent newspaper account: "Jiang Yujie, a transport worker in Shenyang, was cursed and beaten by her husband and mother-in-law after she gave birth to a daughter. Her mother-in-law urged her husband to seek a divorce and promised to find him a wife who could produce a son. Last April, Miss Jiang killed herself by drinking seven bottles of insecticide."

RELIGIOUS INFLUENCES

Oriental attitudes toward suicide are also discussed in detail by Dublin (1963). He points, in particular, to the prevalence of suicide in countries where Buddhism has popular following. Despite the apparent Buddhist prohibition of suicide, ie, that man is obligated to live out his span of life, Buddhism is a religion of resignation and despair which tends to encourage suicide, a clear contradiction. Mohammedanism, on the other hand, in contrast to the other religions of the East, has always condemned suicide with utmost severity in every conceivable circumstance. Suicide is expressly forbidden in the Koran.

Neither the Old nor the New Testament contains any specific prohibition of suicide, but throughout the Old Testament runs the theme of the sacredness of life. Josephus, a historian of the first century of the Christian era, tells that in Judea the body of a suicide was not buried until after sunset, and then it was carried to the grave without the usual burial rites (Guernsey, 1883). Apparently, this is the first explicit Jewish condemnation of the act. With such emphasis on the value of life, it is not strange that religious Jews have always considered suicide a deadly sin. This probably explains the fact that suicide has been extremely rare until very recently among Jews (Dublin, 1963).

In the ethic of early Western society, such as Greece and Rome, suicide was tolerated. However, with the advent of Christianity, it was looked upon as a sin and even murder (Veith, 1969). Hirsh (1960) states that "in medieval society the suicide was treated legally as a murder, his naked body carried through the streets to be buried at a crossroad with a stake driven through his heart."

LANGUAGE AND ETHICAL DERIVATION

The consideration of suicide as murder also has roots in language. For instance, the German word for suicide is Selbastmord or self-murder, which was not found in that language until the 17th century, although the English, from the time of Chaucer, used the phrase "to murder oneself" (Daube, 1977). In an elegant treatise on the linguistics of suicide, Daube considers the relationship of language to the cultural and religious attitudes toward suicide in general.

It was only in the 19th century that suicide was no longer looked upon as the sin of murder, but came to be considered a psychiatric illness and its relationship to the law became a point of ethics (Silving, 1957; Dublin, 1963). In most societies now, a survivor of a suicide attempt is not punished but is treated as psychiatrically ill.

CHAPTER 4

OVERVIEW OF DEMOGRAPHIC AND STATISTICAL FACTORS

GEORGE J. KLEINER
WILMA MARKUS GRESTON

In an effort to obtain data on suicide in association with pregnancy, the only meaningful observations that could be obtained were from cumulative studies of national or large urban population groups. Even those were few in number. Statistical analyses on suicide in association with pregnancy were not readily available, and it was difficult to compare reports because of the immense social, religious, ethnic, cultural, regional, and temporal differences. Those statistical reports that were available were often incomplete, lacking one or more items of standard data, such as age, parity, method of suicide, or duration of pregnancy. In addition, they did not necessarily differentiate between all female suicides and women of childbearing age. Even if only women of childbearing age were included, the age ranges varied. Inconsistencies also included variations as to what constituted the postpartum period, as times from six weeks to 12 months were reported. While it is necessary to accept available statistics, one should be aware of their serious limitations and the difficulties in collecting data on suicide in the general population, as well as the conflicting attitudes on the accuracy of suicide reporting as a whole.

VARIABILITY AND RELIABILITY OF DATA COLLECTION

In writing on the social meaning of suicide, Douglas (1967) contended that official statistics on its incidence are inaccurate to the point of being useless. They are invalid for research purposes because national definitions of suicide differ and because coroners' definitions and search, and ascertainment procedures of suicide differ as well. He felt that, in the face of such obstacles, no conclusions about national, district, and social differences in suicide could be usefully drawn.

In 1968, studies on the comparability of suicide rates were started by the World Health Organization. A questionnaire on procedures for the ascertainment of suicide was sent to interested persons in 24 countries. In its review of the results of that study, *Suicide and Attempted Suicide* (World Health Organization, 1974), the *WHO Chronicle* (1975) article points out that, in most places, an unnatural death was considered accidental until proved a suicide. There was no uniform way of dealing statistically with deaths that were "probably" suicides as they were added in sometimes with suicides and sometimes with accidental deaths or deaths due to unknown causes. Of the 24 participating countries, only Israel gave the number of probable suicides in its national statistics. In most of the countries represented, the police, whose training for this work varied, were responsible for reporting a death from unnatural causes and for collecting evidence from relatives, witnesses, and doctors. It was often thought desirable not to arrive at a suicide verdict, so that the deceased might be buried with full religious rights, the relatives might not be left with feelings of guilt, and the family might not lose life-insurance benefits. It was felt that "doctors, who often must work with probabilities rather than with certainties, and whose pronouncements are not generally disputed, may report a death as suicide with less hesitation than a legal expert who is used to accepting nothing less than complete certainty." An autopsy, an important contribution to the medical evidence, was requested in some places only when suicide was already suspected. Different statistics might result if autopsies were done routinely in all cases of violent or sudden death.

In addition to the difficulties encountered when comparing statistics between countries, long-accepted national statistical characteristics may be rendered invalid on critical review. In a letter to the editor of the *British Medical Journal*, B.M. Barraclough (1974) pointed out that, for 70 years, the Scottish suicide rate had been reported to be lower than for England. He suggested that the difference may be an artifact as the result of differing ascertainment procedures. In fact, he argued that, on review of the corrected figures, the incidence of suicide may be greater in Scotland than in England.

Even more to the point was a report by Atkinson et al (1975) on a study of deaths due to a single causative factor (poisoning) in relatively similar communities in England and Wales. Inconsistencies in suicide ascertainment criteria were suggested, as there were considerable variations among coroners' districts as to the relative proportions of these deaths judged to be suicide or accident.

The high rate of suicide in the Scandinavian countries focused again on the differences of reporting between countries. Pokorny (1973) felt that the differences in the rate of suicides might be the direct result of the type of reporting. He reexamined the observation that suicides were typically high in Denmark and Sweden and typically low in Norway, even though these three countries seemed otherwise similar. He found that there were significantly higher rates of unclassified and accidental deaths in Norway than in Denmark or Sweden. This could account for the reported differences in suicide rates, if one assumed that many of these accidental and unclassified deaths were suicides.

Similar reservations on the accuracy of suicide reporting in Canada were voiced by J.H. Brown (1975). He felt that sustained and systematic efforts to upgrade the quality of reporting were needed as the conclusions of his study lent strong support for the belief that underreporting of suicide in Canada might be considerable. Yet the differences in rates of suicide between the various provinces might be real.

In common with other nations, the United States relies primarily on coroners' offices for suicide reporting. The coroner is generally charged with the official responsibility for certifying the mode of death when unnatural causes are suspected.

In their inquiry into the validity of reported sucide rates in 11 western states of the United States, Nelson et al (1978) found extensive variation in the backgrounds, professional resources, operating procedures, and governing statutes of coroners and coroners' offices and in policies concerning suicide. They suggested that the rates of suicide and the supposedly well-researched relationships between sociodemographic variables could be better understood by controlling for variations in the coroners' offices and their certification processes.

It is likely that reporting on suicide in association with pregnancy is even less reliable, as it might be referred to as maternal death without specifying suicide. This might be done in order not to imply self-destruction in an effort to avoid the family further pain or embarrassment. Similarly, suicide in the early months of pregnancy with only minimal uterine enlargement may be missed by the coroner if inadequate postmortem is done. On the other hand, in cases where the cause of death is clear, a postmortem may not be done; these cases might also be lost to statistical recording because the menstrual history was unknown and a history of pregnancy was unavailable.

In his sociological and statistical study of suicide, Dublin (1963) reported information from a personal communication with Louis Weiner, statistician of the New York City Health Department: "A recent study by the statisticians of the New York City Health Department of deaths from barbiturate poisoning, inhalation of gases, and falls from high places, all under unspecified circumstances, suggested that the recorded suicide figures are understated by as much as one fourth to one third." These errors in data collection must be at least as significant for suicide during pregnancy. In New York City, reporting of suicide is done by the Office of the Medical Examiner. It is our understanding that the medical examiner is not required to report that a woman who committed suicide was pregnant (Freida Nelson, Assistant Director, Bureau of Health Statistics and Analysis, New York City Department of Health, personal communication, 1982). However, this alone could not explain the remarkably low incidence of suicide during pregnancy in New York City which will be discussed further on in this chapter.

As part of her study on methods of suicide, Goodwin (Chapter 8) discusses the accuracy of suicide reporting in New Mexico. She points to instances where death had originally been ruled as accidental or was subsequently judged a suicide in which pregnancy or postpartum status was not determined. Of the 47 suicides, two were pseudo-pregnant, two were pregnant, and two were within the first year postpartum. In addition, she found one case intrapartum and one case postpartum, both of which had not originally been reported as suicides. Thus, of eight cases where Dr. Goodwin did in-depth evaluations, only two were accurately reported as both a suicide and as pregnant on the death certificate.

In addition to the above reports on the "reliability" of official suicide rates, there have been arguments by sociologists and medical writers who advocated that the scientific method could not appropriately be applied to the study of suicide. In particular, official mortality figures were considered worthless as a valid source of information about suicide. Peter Sainsbury (1973) disputed this in his President's Address to the Section of Psychiatry of the Royal Society of Medicine. He stated that suicide reporting has "a privileged status among mortality figures because they are more extensive in scope and in detail than those available on any other deviant form of human behaviour; in England, for instance, records cover more than 150 years." He maintained that the different groups might be compared, trends studied, and the ecology of suicide explored. It might be possible to identify those social groups more or less at risk, note some of the possible causes and common denominators, and seek ways of preventing suicide.

Sainsbury (1973) agreed that suicide was underreported, but he contended that "for all practical, epidemiological purposes, underreporting or seeking the absolute rate of suicide is of small consequence." He argued rather vigorously that "what matters, and what the epidemiologist needs to establish clearly, is whether the differences he observes between the rates of particular social, clinical or other categories are valid." Sainsbury (1973) maintained that "countries really do differ in their incidence of suicide in spite of their different ways of defining or reporting it" and "that it is not reporting but variations in social ecology which are accounting for regional differences in suicide."

He reasserted this view in a more recent article on the accuracy of officially reported suicide statistics for purposes of epidemiologic research (Sainsbury and Jenkins, 1982). After analyzing the underreporting of suicides and the reliability of official rates which are subject to error from variations in defining and reporting cases, they concluded that these sources of error did not invalidate the differences found between cultural and social groups because they were randomized, at least to an extent that would allow epidemiologists to compare rates among countries, districts, demographic groups, and over time.

This view was also supported by Barraclough (1973). In this study, one of several of his on the underreporting of suicide, he used the World Health Organization's new mortality category of "undetermined deaths" to obtain a combined rate with suicide in comparing 22 countries. His conclusions suggested that national inconsistencies about defining suicide do not account for national differences in its incidence.

Despite the obvious differences in the mechanics of data collection on suicide in general and the ambiguity as to their value, it is necessary to use whatever reports are available to rationally evaluate the incidence of suicide. These problems are multiplied many-fold when attempts are made to obtain statistical data specifically on suicide in association with pregnancy (Barno, 1967; OSMA Committee on Maternal Health, 1966, 1976; Arthure, 1968; Goodhart, 1968; Resnik and Wittlin, 1971; New York City Department of Health, 1983; Goodwin, Chapter 8).

This chapter attempts to collate available data in a comprehensive manner. It reflects a thorough search of available literature in an effort to determine the possible incidence of suicide during pregnancy with some accuracy. The data have been standardized, whenever possible, in order to compile the statistics from a multitude of sources, with their inherent differences, into tabular form for comparison. In the following material, the definition of suicide during pregnancy generally includes only the duration of pregnancy and three months postpartum, to coincide with the New York City definition. Other reports have included women who attempted or committed suicide up to one year or more postpartum. Whenever possible, from the description of data reported by others, we have limited the cumulative statistics to reports of women who were no more than three months postpartum, unless otherwise noted. It was not possible to set limits on another variable, the women's reproductive age. Some reports recorded incidence of suicide during pregnancy against a control of women of childbearing age up to age 45, others to age 49. As the incidence of pregnancy is very low between ages 45 and 49, raising the age limit will artificially decrease the rate of suicide during pregnancy.

STATISTICS ON SUICIDE DURING PREGNANCY

Early Surveys

Table 4-1 is a composite of figures from various central and eastern European countries with data collected approximately to the end of World War II. It should be noted that the total number of cases was relatively small. In these surveys, of the 1766 women suicides reviewed, 222

Table 4-1
Early Surveys of Women Suicides

Source	Year of Publication	Women Suicides	Number Pregnant	Percent
Heller	1900	70	7	10
Ollendorf	1905	49	1	2
Pilcz	1905	211	56	26.5
Pfeiffer	1912	141	9	6.4
Mosdzien	1926	33	1	3
Sachwitz	1927	46	6	13
Elo	1931	187	18	9.6
Babin	1933	20	3	15
Krugelstein	1936	107	0	0
Beitzke	1938	91	12	13.2
Pilcz	1940	428	85	19.8
Dahlgren	1945	136	5	3.7
Bengtsson	1947	247	19	7.7
Total		1766	222	12.6

Modified after Bengtsson, 1947; McClure et al, 1971.

or 12.6% were pregnant and the incidence of suicide in pregnancy varied from zero to 26.5% of women suicides as a whole. However, the women's ages were not specified. Studies cited by McClure et al (1971) included women up to age 50, and it is possible that in some reports quoted by Bengtsson (1947) females beyond the extremes of childbearing age had been included, possibly making the suicide rate falsely low.

Current Surveys

Completed suicide A detailed search of the literature of the past three decades on the incidence of suicide in association with pregnancy was undertaken. An effort was made to gather all surveys and individual case reports. It is possible that some case reports may have been missed because the title of the article was not specific enough or was oriented to a different aspect of medicine. Because statistics had not been gathered in a uniform manner, in order to compare reports, the incidence of suicide during pregnancy will be approached in three ways, ie, the percentage of pregnant females who committed suicide out of the total number of suicides of women of childbearing age, the percentage of maternal deaths which were due to suicide, and the rate of suicides during pregnancy in relation to total maternities of a given location.

Published surveys of suicides which included pregnant women revealed that only 119 women or 1.8% were pregnant when they committed suicide, out of a total of 6454 women suicides of childbearing age (Table 4-2). It may seem incongruous to list the study by Sim (1963) which reported zero incidence of suicide during pregnancy and those of

Table 4-2
Recent Surveys of Suicides in Women of Childbearing Age

Source	Inclusive Years of Study	No. of Suicides	Number Pregnant	Percent
Ribeiro, 1962 Nairobi, Kenya	1958–60	26	2	7.7
Höök, 1963 Sweden	1947–50	100	5	5
Sim, 1963 Birmingham, England	1950–56	119	0	0
Heiman, 1965	—	300	4	1.3
Potondi, 1965 Budapest, Hungary	4 years	326	11	3.4
Rosen, cited by Resnik and Wittlin, 1965 Maryland, USA	—	700	1*	0.1
Seagar and Flood, 1965 Bristol, England	1957–61	43	3	7
Heller and Whittington, 1968 Denver, Colorado, USA	1967	38	1*	2.6
Resnik and Wittlin, 1971 Miami, Minneapolis, Rochester, Philadelphia, USA	1968–69	202	1	0.5
Eungprubhanth, 1975 Bangkok, Thailand	1960–69	197†	11	5.6
Price and Karim, 1975 Fiji Islands	1971–72	16	2	12.5
Dept. of Health, 1983 New York City, USA	1961–80	2437	6	0.25
Weir‡ London, England	1943–62	1696	66	3.9
Goodwin§ New Mexico, USA	1974–76	47	3	6.4
Rosenberg‖ California, USA	1961–63	207	3	1.4
Total		6454	119	1.8

*In the memory of the chief medical examiner (Rosen study), chief pathologist (Heller and Whittington study).
†Up to age 40 only.
‡See Chapter 5.
§See Chapter 8.
‖See Chapter 9.

Rosen (1965) and Heller and Whittington (1968) because the one suicide listed in each was only in the memory of the person keeping records. They have been included because these reports were of studies which specifically attempted to identify suicide in association with pregnancy and where virtually none was found. It should be noted that most of the reports in Table 4-2 that contained small samples of women, ie, those with less than 50 women suicides (Ribeiro, 1962; Seagar and Flood, 1965; Price and Karim, 1975; Goodwin, Chapter 8) were associated with the highest percent of suicides during pregnancy.

The substantial differences in statistics in the years before and after World War II are interesting, ie, 12.6% versus 1.8% or a sevenfold decrease (Table 4-3). Perhaps it is possible to explain these differences by considering that family planning, legalization and availability of abortion, and improvement in education and the standard of living have become almost universal for the countries reported. It is generally recognized that there also has been a concomitant relaxation of religious and moral scruples and greater sexual awareness and freedoms. These have, perhaps, resulted in a better self-image by the woman and lessened her internal frustrations in association with pregnancy.

It is difficult to understand the differences found among reports from large urban or industrial centers in Great Britain. Sim (1963) reported on 119 women suicides, quoting information from the coroner of the city of Birmingham (England). None were pregnant, although in two cases the woman thought she might be pregnant, but this was not confirmed by medical or postmortem examination. In fact, the coroner made a statement that, for 1950 to 1956, "We have no record of any woman known to be pregnant having committed suicide." Weir* reported on 1696 completed suicides in London for the years 1943 to 1962; 66 women or 4% were pregnant. Seagar and Flood (1965) reported on 43 suicides in Bristol; three women or 7% were pregnant. Based on the figures from London and Bristol, one would have expected Birmingham to have had from five to eight suicides, and yet there were none, despite social, cultural, religious, and demographic similarities in the population. Perhaps regional differences must be considered more seriously.

Equally intriguing are the marked differences between the two large metropolitan centers of New York City and London. Of 2437 female suicides in New York City between 1961 and 1980, six women or 0.25% were pregnant. For the sake of comparison, if one extrapolated from the London figures, the expected number of suicides in New York City would have been 97. It is hard to find an explanation for only six suicides found when 97 were expected and for why these two large cities, with much in common, should be so dramatically different. It might be possi-

*A detailed analysis and discussion can be found in Chapter 5.

Table 4-3
Surveys of Women Suicides Before and After World War II

Years	Number of Suicides	Number Pregnant	Percent
1900–1947	1766	222	12.6
1943–1980	6454	119	1.8

ble that the inclusive years reported, ie, 1943 to 1962 in London versus 1961 to 1980 in New York City, during which time the abortion laws changed in the latter, might account for some of the differences. Also, the postpartum period is considered to be one year for statistical purposes in England, but is only three months in New York City.

As far back as the fifties in New York City, the incidence of suicide during pregnancy was apparently very low also. During a discussion on other aspects of the abortion problem at a Planned Parenthood conference on abortion in 1958, McLane stated that the incidence of suicide in women of childbearing age (14–50) is about the same as in the total female population, 5.5 per 100,000. In 1953 in New York City the incidence of suicide among pregnant women was 0.55 per 100,000 or 1/10 of the rate of all women of childbearing age.

Having been associated with three large maternity services over a 25-year period and more than 200,000 deliveries, the senior author knew of only one clearly identified case of suicide during pregnancy. This, in fact, served as the impetus for this work. It is our intuitive feeling that this extreme rarity of suicide during pregnancy in New York City is reasonably accurate.

Resnik and Wittlin (1971) also attest to the rarity of suicide in association with pregnancy in their survey of female suicides from four major metropolitan areas of the United States—Miami, Minneapolis, Rochester, and Philadelphia. Of 202 recorded suicides in women between the ages of 13 and 50 on which autopsy was performed, only one (0.5%) was pregnant.

The differences between the states of New Mexico and California and the New York City figures also stand out. In New Mexico, Goodwin (Chapter 8) reported on 47 suicides of whom three (6.4%) were pregnant. Rosenberg (Chapter 9) reported on 207 suicides, of whom three (1.4%) were pregnant. The incidence of suicide during pregnancy in each state was markedly different, and each was considerably higher than that reported for New York City. Again, regional variations might account for some of these differences, but one must suspect that reporting methods could play a significant role as well.

Another way to look at the incidence of suicide in pregnancy is to establish what percentage of maternal deaths are due to suicide. The maternal death rate or mortality is the number of maternal deaths per

100,000 live births that occur as the direct result of the reproductive process. Maternal mortality is given only for purely obstetrical complications in the United States Vital Statistics and does not include associated causes. However, in the British reports (Reports on Confidential Enquiries into Maternal Deaths in England and Wales), maternal deaths are recorded as due to purely obstetrical causes ("true" maternal deaths) as well as to those in association with diseases occurring in the presence of pregnancy. The Reports on Confidential Enquiries into Maternal Deaths in England and Wales showed that approximately two thirds of all maternal deaths were associated with purely obstetrical complications and the remaining one third with associated causes such as heart, liver, and kidney diseases. When reviewing the incidence of suicide in pregnancy, one should look for deaths listed both ways.

During a nine-year period in England and Wales (Report on Confidential Enquiries into Maternal Deaths in England and Wales, 1967–1975), there were 1045 "true" maternal deaths. Of these, 53 were suicides during pregnancy, labor, delivery, and the first year postpartum or one suicide for every 20 "true" maternal deaths (5%). If, however, one excluded the postpartum period, the number of women who killed themselves while pregnant was 18 or one suicide for every 58 "true" maternal deaths (1.7%).

In the United States as a whole, the total maternal mortality for 1978 (United States Vital Statistics, 1982) was 324 women who died from purely obstetrical causes. But there was no information identifying those women who might have died by suicide. In some states, special committees reviewed maternal mortality; occasionally, suicide was singled out. The Committee on Maternal Death of the Ohio State Medical Association (1966) stated that "in a period of 9 years (1955–1963) there were approximately 1025 maternal deaths. In 10 of the cases the cause of death is related to suicide associated with the pregnancy state."

Using the most current data, ie, compiled statistics from 1978 (United States Vital Statistics, 1982), the number of maternal deaths was 324 and the total number of live births was 3,338,300, an incidence of approximately 10 per 100,000 live births in the United States. This is a significant reduction from 36 per 100,000 live births in 1963, when suicide during pregnancy was first reviewed by the authors. If a completed suicide in pregnancy represents 1% of maternal deaths, as Heiman (1965) suggested, and as maternal deaths in the United States occur at the rate of 10 per 100,000 live births, then the anticipated incidence of suicide in pregnancy would be 0.1 per 100,000 or 1 per million live births. To put it another way, considering the 3.5 million live births (approximately) which occur annually, the expected total number of completed suicides of pregnant women in the United States should be less than four women per year.

One other way to look at the reality of suicide during pregnancy and postpartum is to consider its frequency in relation to total maternities. In England, detailed reports into maternal deaths, which began in 1952, are gathered triannually (Report on Confidential Enquiries into Maternal Deaths in England and Wales, 1952–1954; 1955–1957; 1958–1960; 1961–1963; 1964–1966; 1967–1969; 1970–1972; 1973–1975). Even though some information regarding 21 deaths ascribed to suicide in pregnancy were mentioned for 1956–1966, until 1967 they "had no knowledge of actual number of deaths from suicide related to pregnancy or childbirth, because previously in such cases the fact of pregnancy was usually omitted from the death certificate" (Report on Confidential Enquiries into Maternal Deaths in England and Wales, 1967–1969). In the nine-year period 1967–1975, there were 6,677,211 "maternities," ie, the number of women who gave birth to one or more registered live or stillborn babies. The rate of suicide during pregnancy and postpartum was 1 per 125,985 maternities (Table 4-4). When considering the antepartum period alone, during which approximately one third of the suicides reported took place, the suicide rate was 1 per 370,956 maternities.

The one major report from the United States which is comparable to the confidential enquiries in recording deaths from suicide against "maternities" is that of Barno (1967). The only minor difference is that the statistics were given for live births only. In Barno's (1967) report from the Minnesota Maternal Mortality Committee for a 16-year period (1950–1965), there were 14 maternal suicides among 1,301,745 live births, an incidence of 1 in 92,982 (Table 4-4). Ten of these occurred postpartum and four with fetus in utero.

Thus, the incidence of death during pregnancy and the postpartum period, as reported from Minnesota, was approximately 1 in 100,000 if one considered deaths for one year postpartum and approximately 1 in 300,000 during pregnancy alone. It is also of interest to note from Table

Table 4-4
Incidence of Suicide during Pregnancy in Relation to Total Births

		Suicides		Incidence	
Source	Total Births*	*Total*†	*During Pregnancy Only*	*Total*†	*During Pregnancy Only*
Barno (1967)	1,301,745	14	4	1/92,982	1/325,436
England and Wales‡	6,677,211	53	18	1/125,985	1/370,956

*See text for explanation.
†During pregnancy and up to 1 year postpartum.
‡Reports on Confidential Enquiries into Maternal Deaths in England and Wales (1969–1975).

4-4 that, despite national differences between Minnesota and England and Wales and the years during which the data was collected, the incidence of both total suicides (during pregnancy and up to one year postpartum) and suicides during pregnancy alone were very similar. If one were to consider the incidence of suicide during pregnancy against the total number of maternities in the United States, which is approximately 3.5 million annually, then the expected number of maternal deaths due to suicide in pregnancy alone should be not more than 10 women per year.

An attempt has been made to establish the frequency of completed suicide among pregnant women in the United States. Considered from the background of maternal mortality, the anticipated number should be less than four per year. From the number extrapolated from total maternities, not more than 10 women per year would be expected to commit suicide. Thus, in reality, the projected number of women who will die due to suicide in pregnancy should be between four and 10 per year. A small number indeed.

Yet, as this material was being analyzed, two reports were headlined in the *New York Daily News*. One was a 14-year-old schoolgirl, nine months pregnant, who stepped in front of a train as a deliberate act of suicide (Darkness at Noon, 1983). Within a few weeks, there was another report of a mother plunging to her death after drowning her 12-day-old baby (Fay and Meskil, 1983). It is obvious that, with such small numbers of suicides during pregnancy, individual cases such as these can markedly affect the statistical data. However, it is still unlikely that a physician will encounter this problem directly during his or her professional life.

Attempted suicide Some reports in the literature identify attempted suicide in pregnancy as a major topic; others include pregnant women in the discussion of attempted suicide as a whole. These reports have been compiled for comparison (Table 4-5). It was not always possible to assess with accuracy what percentage of women were of childbearing age. Therefore, it is likely that some of the numbers were a reflection of all women suicides. Of the total of 2681 women, 176 or 6.6% attempted suicide while pregnant. The incidence of attempted suicide during pregnancy taken from the compiled data ranged from 3% to 22%. If one compares the incidence of completed suicide during pregnancy (1. 8% in Table 4-2) with the incidence of attempted suicide (6.6% in Table 4-5), it appears that attempted suicide is at least 3½ times more frequent. It is particularly important to note that attempted suicide in the postpartum period is probably not reflected in these statistics. It is also possible that the incidence is artificially low because a number of women who attempt suicide in early pregnancy may not admit to being pregnant (Otto, 1972).

While these figures might be true as a reflection of attempted suicide in the population as a whole, they appear to the authors to be grossly

Table 4-5
Surveys of Attempted Suicides in Women of Childbearing Age

Source	No. of Attempted Suicides	Number Pregnant	Percent
Schmidt et al, 1955 Missouri, USA	60	2*	3.3
Epps, 1957 England	100	8	8
Harrington and Cross, 1959 England	33	6	18.2
James et al, 1963 Australia	56*	5	8.9
Sclare and Hamilton, 1963 Scotland	103	5	4.9
Taylor et al, 1964 England	100	3	3
Jacobziner, 1965 New York City, USA	448	22*	4.9
Boxall and Chauvel, 1966 Australia	57*	4*	7
Burke, 1968 England	58	7	12.1
Otto, 1972† Sweden	1226	75	6.1
Burke, 1976 Birmingham, England	41	9	22
Whitlock‡ Australia	399	30	7.5
Total	2681	176	6.6

*Extrapolated from numbers or percentages given in report.
†Follow-up of 1965 study.
‡See Chapter 6.

underreported. In one year at Montefiore Medical Center, North Central Bronx Hospital (NCB) in New York City, there were four women who attempted suicide admitted on an obstetrical service which delivers 2500 women per year. In addition, their adolescent service has seen seven pregnant teen-agers who attempted suicide during the past four years. In New York City, management of obstetrical patients takes place primarily in outpatient clinics or in private physicians' offices. If a suicide attempt takes place which is serious enough to warrant hospital admission, the woman may be housed on an obstetrical floor, not necessarily on a psychiatric unit, although a psychiatrist would be called in for consultation.

This is probably true for most other teaching hospitals in the United States as well. In such a situation, the woman might escape statistical analysis as most suicide data is obtained from psychiatrists or from psychiatric hospitals. The number of suicide attempts noted at NCB alone is remarkably high when contrasted with the six completed suicides in pregnant women in New York City over a 19-year period (New York City Department of Health, 1983, Table 4-2). From our experience, it appears that the spread between the incidence of attempted suicide and completed suicide in pregnant women may be much greater than the 3½-fold difference that has been gathered from the literature.

Parity

A possible relationship between parity and completed suicide during pregnancy is worth mentioning, although most large studies do not detail this information. The only report containing a substantial number of suicides during pregnancy which included details of parity is that of Weir (Chapter 5). It can be seen in Figure 4-1 that primiparous women predominate as compared to subsequent individual parities. Fifty-eight percent of the women committed suicide during their first pregnancy, which is not unexpected as primiparous women are the single largest group giving birth. However, this is somewhat higher than the 30–40% of primip-

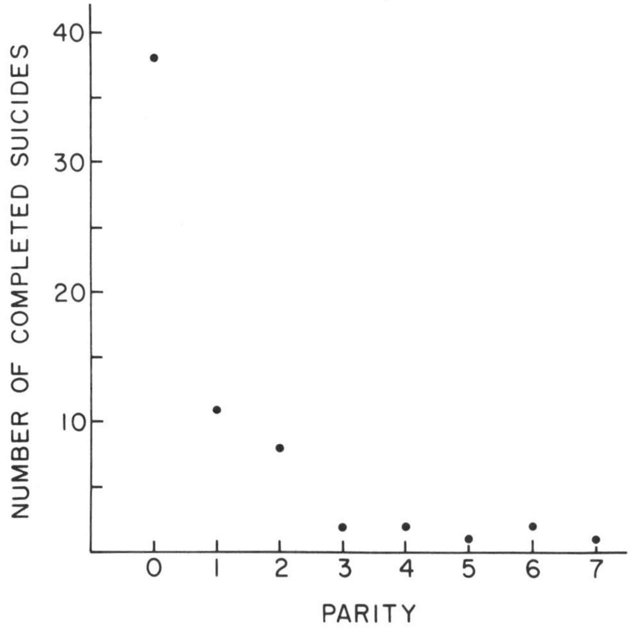

Figure 4-1 Suicide during pregnancy by parity (modified from Weir, Chapter 5).

arous deliveries seen currently in the United States. Without attempting to overinterpret, one must assume from these data that a primiparous woman is more likely to commit suicide while pregnant than is a multiparous one.

Marital Status

It appears that being unmarried (single, widowed, separated, or divorced) may have some impact on suicide attempts and on the completed act of suicide during pregnancy and the puerperium (Table 4-6). Completed suicide in relation to marital status was reviewed by two authors. In a Swedish study on pregnancy and suicide, of 19 women who committed suicide, only one was married (Bengtsson, 1947). Weir (Chapter 5) reviewed London figures which showed that there appeared to be no difference between the suicide rates of pregnant or nonpregnant women if married (38.5% vs 41.5%). Similarly, there were no differences in the unmarried group (61.5% vs 57.9%, respectively). However, among those women who committed suicide while pregnant, 61.5% were unmarried whereas only 38.5% were married. In attempted suicide, Whitlock and Edwards (1968) found that marital status had no influence on its incidence in pregnant and nonpregnant women in Australia. In threatened suicide, it appears that marital status might be a provoking

Table 4-6
Marital Status and Suicide

		Married (%)		Unmarried* (%)	
Source	*Type of Suicide*	*Pregnant*	*Non-pregnant*	*Pregnant*	*Non-pregnant*
Bengtsson, 1947 Sweden	Completed	1	—	18	—
Weir† London	Completed	38.5	41.4	61.5	57.9
Whitlock and Edwards, 1968 Australia	Attempted	47	58	53	52
Medical Board, 1953‡ Sweden	Threatened	8	—	48	—
Inghe, 1944 Sweden	Threatened	2	—	10	—

*Single, widowed, divorced, separated.
†See Chapter 5.
‡Reference: SOU 1953/29.

factor. Two studies from Sweden indicated that more unmarried than married women threatened to commit suicide in their application for permission for abortion. The data was collected at a time when abortion in Sweden could be obtained only by applying to the medical board. Inghe (1944) reviewed figures from the years 1933–1941 from the National Association for Sexual Information; 10 of the pregnant women were unmarried, only two were married. The Swedish Medical Board figures published in 1953 (SOU 1953/29) indicated that of 56 women who threatened suicide, 48 were unmarried.

Marital status may also have some impact on when during the pregnancy suicide is most likely to occur. Weir's (Chapter 5) figures show that in early pregnancy (4–16 weeks) suicide occurred in six married and 24 unmarried women. In the latter part of pregnancy (17–40 weeks) the distribution was relatively even, with 19 married and 16 unmarried women committing suicide. It appears, therefore, that in completed and threatened suicide, being single may be a contributing factor to the incidence and timing of suicide in pregnancy.

An editorial in the *British Medical Journal* (Suicide Risk in Teenage Pregnancy, 1971) offered further thoughts on possible correlations between marital status and suicide. It pointed out that "since Emile Durkheim's classic studies it has been recognized that married people and parents are less likely to commit suicide than unmarried or childless people." The editorial also mentioned Evans (1967), who had drawn attention to the apparent paradox of very high rates of self-poisoning in married women under the age of 20. Perhaps it is age, rather than marital status, that may be a more significant causative factor associated with suicide during pregnancy.

Teen-age Pregnancy

Suicide risk in teen-age pregnancy deserves special mention. It appears that there may be a higher risk of attempted and even completed suicide in the young pregnant woman. In recent times, the pregnant teen-ager has become a frequent subject of concern in our society, as teen-age pregnancy, especially in large urban centers in the United States, has assumed epidemic proportions (When Children Bear Children, 1983). The pregnant teen-ager is socially and emotionally handicapped and also may be prone to a variety of medical complications of pregnancy. Since many authorities consider teen-age pregnancy to be a part of acting out and a signal for attention and need of support, it is possible that threatened, attempted, and even completed suicide may be an extension of this abnormal behavior.

Writing in the *American Journal of Psychotherapy* on current trends in suicidal behavior in the United States, Frederick (1978) stated that while the overall suicide rate continues to increase, the most striking upturn could be seen in both sexes between the ages of 15 and 20. The increase among females in the younger age ranges was 128%. Of especially serious concern was the dramatic rise in the suicide rate between the ages of 10 and 14. However, other than sporadic case reports, the literature had no studies on completed suicide in pregnant teen-agers, but mainly discussed threats and attempted suicide.

In 1971, a *British Medical Journal* editorial (Suicide Risk in Teenage Pregnancy, 1971) stated that "pregnancy in young patients is associated with distinct hazards," whether married or unmarried. It noted that there are special obstetric and psychologic risks in teen-age pregnancy. They argued forcefully that suicide in association with pregnancy in teen-agers is not a myth, but a serious reality. Otto (1972), in his follow-up study of attempted suicide among 1226 girls and women under 21 years of age, stated that 75 or 6.1% were pregnant. Sixty of them were teen-agers, and the youngest of those pregnant was 14 years old. The relatively high number of attempted suicides seen in the adolescent clinic at NCB (see Attempted Suicide in this chapter) points to the need for particular vigilance among pregnant teen-agers. It may be of interest to note that one of the recent cases of completed suicide in pregnancy, previously mentioned as headlined in the *Daily News* (Darkness at Noon, 1983), was that of a 14-year-old girl from Maryland who stepped in front of a train. Yet, paradoxically, in the authors' experience, many pregnant adolescents are generally happy to continue with pregnancy despite social and family pressures to the contrary. Many vigorously refuse abortion.

Gabrielson (Chapter 11) discussed 105 pregnant teen-agers, 17 years of age or younger, who were admitted to the Yale-New Haven Hospital for delivery over a two-year period. The study revealed that 14 of the young mothers were subsequently known to have made one or more self-destructive attempts or threats which were serious enough to require care or to be reported to the physician at the hospital. They concluded that teen-age pregnancy may have a direct effect on the future potential for suicidal behavior.

CHAPTER 5

SUICIDE DURING PREGNANCY IN LONDON: 1943–1962

J.G. WEIR

THE MATERIAL

This chapter is about the women who committed suicide while pregnant in London Administrative County during the 20 years from 1943 to 1962. London Administrative County, or London AC, consists of the 28 metropolitan boroughs and the City of London. The population was about 3.25 million and the mean annual number of live births was some 55,000. The material was obtained from the depositions of H.M. Coroners for London. In England, it is established practice that doctors inform the coroner of any death caused by poisoning, accident, injury, abortion, or in which the cause is not clear. Then there is an additional screening, ie, the registrar of deaths is legally obliged to inform the coroner when he suspects that death is associated with unnatural causes or when he has reason to believe that the cause is unknown.

It may be safely assumed that every cause of suicide during pregnancy was reported to the coroner. In recent years, concern has been expressed about suicidal deaths from drug overdose which are wrongly certified as due to natural causes (Patel, 1974). But when this happens, it is among elderly people. A pregnant suicide might not have been known to be pregnant when her death was reported, it might not have been thought that she had committed suicide, and a verdict of suicide might not have been recorded at the end of the coroner's inquiry; but all sudden deaths of women in the fertile years were sure to have been reported to him. "Any death of which the cause is unknown may be unnatural and should be reported," wrote one of the coroners who kindly allowed me access to their depositions. "Sudden death in a previously healthy woman of childbearing age, for instance, is unlikely to be from natural causes. The only common natural disaster that occurs in this group is rupture of an aneurysm of the circle of Willis. Such deaths must always be approached with suspicion, since they may be due to abortion or barbiturate poisoning" (Thurston, 1967).

It may also be accepted that pregnancies of four weeks' duration onwards were always detected. An autopsy was performed in all cases, even in those where death appeared to be due to multiple injuries, and the uterus was routinely examined. I inquired about this before I began the investigation from the three forensic pathologists who performed autopsies for the coroners, and they answered firmly in the affirmative. This was confirmed in their reports. There was generally some mention of the uterus—it was normal, it was small or it was large, it contained a fibroid or a polyp, or the endometrium was at a particular phase. When an embryo or a fetus was discovered, the duration of the pregnancy was then established. Generally this was obtained by measurement of the fetus and, in early cases, ovarian histology was employed. In several cases the pathologist's report of a pregnancy came out of the blue, there being no mention of it in the report of the coroner's officer—informative though these reports usually were.

It may not be assumed, however, that every case of suicide was assigned a verdict of suicide. There were cases in which it seems very likely that the woman committed suicide, but an open verdict or even a verdict of accidental death was recorded. The cases of Mrs. C.O. and Mrs. C.N. are illustrative.

Mrs. C.O., 35 weeks pregnant, was keen to have this, her first, child, but for a few weeks she had become increasingly depressed and was worried about having a complicated labor. She was admitted to a psychiatric hospital. Her husband had dinner with her there that evening and the next. On the third evening he could not find her. He drove home, and there she was lying on the kitchen floor with her head resting on the drop-type door of the gas cooker, its shelves having been removed. "She was very houseproud," he said at the inquest, "and I can only assume that she was cleaning the cooker when she was overcome for some reason, fell in front of the cooker and in falling inadvertently turned on the tap." She had said to her husband that she would be better off dead and save him all the worry, but at the inquest he denied having told the coroner's officer this. An open verdict was recorded.

Mrs. C.N., like Mrs. C.O., was aged 32. She was expecting her fourth child in four months' time. She helped her husband to run a public house, but their relationship was becoming increasingly disharmonious. Three times in the past seven months she had terminated quarrels with her husband by a suicide attempt. She had been taken to hospital with a large overdose of phenytoin (she had been epileptic since age 16) and twice she had tried to gas herself. A few days before her death, her doctor thought she was so depressed that she should be admitted to hospital, but the psychiatrist who visited her did not think so. On Christmas Eve they were busy serving drinks. When her husband saw her helping herself, he told her to ease up because they had a long night ahead. This nettled her, and she drank more. In the early hours after they had closed and tidied up, she tried to provoke him but he ignored her. She went up to bed. He had taken to sleeping downstairs because of the acrimony between them. In the morning he found her dead in bed, her room filled with coal gas, a chair wedged against the door. A verdict of accidental death was recorded.

These odd verdicts do not reflect upon the competence of the London coroners, but follow the ruling of English law. A suicide verdict must not be recorded merely because suicide seems to be the likely explanation. Suicide must be proved by evidence, affirmatively proved, and must never be presumed (Jervis, 1957).* This is the law in England, unlike Sweden and Denmark where suicide may be presumed if there is no evidence to the contrary.

In order to uncover all the cases of pregnant suicides concealed behind open verdicts and verdicts of accidental death, I examined all the depositions of women aged 15 to 49. The coroner's officers had prepared reports in all cases, usually admirably thorough, and had often obtained statements from friends, relatives, employers, and doctors of the deceased women. To this I added other information I had been able to collect, although always sparing relatives and friends. A few records nevertheless remained stubbornly meager. The nonsuicide-verdict cases were then divided into those in which suicide was infeasible or unlikely and those which were likely to have been suicides. Indicators such as previous attempts, threats of suicide, psychiatric history, evidence of depression, serious deterioration of social conditions, and other life events were kept in mind. Suicide has its gray area, however, even without legal trammels: "open" or conjectural cases remained. But this group was left as small as possible.

Suicide—infeasible Of these, three were pregnant. Two died from a fire starting in the floor below. The third was a Salvation Army officer, seven months pregnant, who had had a shotgun marriage and wore tight corsets to conceal her pregnancy. She vomited and died from inhalation of her vomitus. The tight corsets were thought to have caused the vomiting. She could have taken an abortifacient. However, she clearly did not commit suicide.

Suicide—unlikely Of these, seven were pregnant. Two were knocked down by a car while carelessly crossing the road and one by a horse-drawn coal trolley. One was knocked off her bicycle by a lorry, one drove her motorcycle into a lorry on her way to work, and one fell with her child from a tramcar. The seventh was a 43-year-old primigravida, 36 weeks pregnant, who died in a fire in her little flat. She was a heavy smoker, sometimes smoked in bed, and may have set fire to her

*This point of law was restated in the Court of Appeals on January 30, 1967 (in David decd.) and again on July 1, 1975 (R.v.H.M. Coroner for the City of London).

bedclothes in this way. For six years she had lived alone in the flat during the week, but usually joined her husband in their suburban house on the weekends. Her husband said she had been living in the flat until suitable town accommodation for them was found.

Conjectural Of these, two were pregnant. One was a 29-year-old married primigravida, six months pregnant. An obstetrician who had treated her first for infertility and then during her pregnancy said she had lately become anxious, and he had prescribed a day-time sedative. "Highly strung, egocentric and hypochondriacal" a medical friend said of her. She had told her husband in the morning that she had had no sleep despite her night sedative. When he returned in the evening, he could not rouse her, and she died in hospital of barbiturate poisoning. The forensic pathologist said that, judging from the barbiturate blood level, she might have taken a strong additional dose in her determination to have a sleep. The other was a 19-year-old single primigravida, three months pregnant, who was struck by an electric train while she stood on the platform. She was Italian and spoke no English. Five days before her death, she had left her hospital domestic work telling a friend her boyfriend would look after her. But he had a wife in Italy and, from his statement, was not very interested in the girl.

There were 1444 cases in which a verdict of suicide was recorded and 53 of these were pregnant; 252 cases were probably suicide, although another verdict was recorded, and 13 of these were pregnant. Thus there was a grand total of 1696 cases, and 66 were pregnant at the time of death. One of these, however, had an early tubal pregnancy and is not included among the pregnant suicides in further considerations.

She was a 27-year-old divorcee. She had called on a general practitioner, a new one for her, six days before her death, and had expressed dissatisfaction over her previous medical attendant. He agreed to take her on his list provided she allowed him to make an appointment with a psychiatrist, for she had made two serious suicide attempts with sleeping pills in the past 13 months. She killed herself with an overdose of barbiturates before she saw the psychiatrist. I wrote to the general practitioner less than a year later and he remembered well the one interview he had with her. He found her a disturbed young woman, but there was no mention of amenorrhea or of abdominal pain.

Two of the pregnant suicides apparently came to London with the express intention of committing suicide.

Miss A.C., 37 weeks pregnant, was a student nurse in a hospital 140 miles north of London. On her day off she came to London and booked in at a hotel near the railway terminus. She had no luggage and said she only intended staying one night. Next morning she was found under the bedclothes, wearing only a slip and a brassiere, dead from coal-gas poisoning.

Mrs. B.W. was a housewife and five months pregnant. For 12 months she had been subject to fits of depression, and she had recently been discharged from hospital appearing much improved. She came to London from her home 26 miles away and jumped off Waterloo Bridge into the Thames.

Some people come to London for the purpose of committing suicide and some Londoners go out of London to commit suicide. There is no information about how many come in or go out or whether the two in any way balance. But these two cases were retained in the pregnant suicide group.

METHODS OF SUICIDE

There were no striking differences between the methods of suicide used by the pregnant women and those used by the women who were not pregnant. The methods are summarized in Table 5-1. When a combination of methods was used, the item which directly caused death was taken. Thus a woman who cut her wrists and threw herself from a high window was classified under "jumping from a height."

Table 5-1
Methods of Suicide Employed by Pregnant and Nonpregnant Suicides

	Pregnant Suicides		Nonpregnant Female Suicides Aged 15–19
Method of Suicide	*Number*	*Percent*	*Percent*
Barbiturate poisoning	13	20.0	22.0
Aspirin poisoning	2	3.1	5.1
Other analgesics and soporifics	2	3.1	2.1
Corrosive poisoning	1	1.5	3.2
Coal-gas poisoning	31	47.7	40.0
Hanging	1	1.5	3.1
Drowning	7	10.8	7.4
Jumping from a height	1	1.5	8.3
Jumping in front of a train	5	7.7	6.1
Setting fire to herself	1	1.5	0.4
Car exhaust fumes	1	1.5	0.0
Cutting throat or wrist	0		0.9
Others	0		0.6
Unknown	0		0.8
Total	65	100	100

Coal-gas poisoning was by far the commonest method, and somewhat more commonly used by the pregnant group. The decline in suicide by domestic gas, because of the introduction of oil-based gas and then natural gas, had not begun in the period examined. Indeed, there were 193 more cases in the second decade than in the first. Ten of the pregnant suicides were reported to have had previously made one or more unsuccessful attempts. There were reports of 231 of the nonpregnant group having had made attempts, a slightly smaller proportion.

INPATIENT PSYCHIATRIC TREATMENT

The pregnant suicides seem to have been mentally healthier than the nonpregnant suicides, if admission for psychiatric treatment is used as an index. Three hundred eighty-one (23%) of the nonpregnant group and six (9%) of the pregnant group were reported to have had inpatient psychiatric treatment. These figures could be misleading because the pregnant women tended to be young, and thus the nonpregnant group is overrepresented at the older end of the 15 to 49 age range—the end where women were more likely to have psychiatric illness. To avoid this, Table 5-2 breaks down to the two groups quinquennially. The pregnant suicide group is still indicated as having been mentally healthier, although less strikingly.

Five of the six pregnant women had been admitted to a psychiatric hospital during their pregnancy, and the pregnancy seemed to play some part in their being admitted. The sixth one had been in a psychiatric hospital before her pregnancy. The psychiatrist whom she continued to see considered her pregnancy was the immediate precipitant of her death.

Miss A.Q., aged 22, was 19 weeks pregnant when she drowned herself. Twelve weeks before, having missed her second period, she turned on the gas in her room at two o'clock in the morning. A neighbor smelled the gas, and she was taken to a general hospital. When she recovered, she

Table 5-2
Prevalence of Previous Inpatient Psychiatric Treatment in Pregnant and Nonpregnant Suicides, Compared by Age

	Pregnant Suicides		Nonpregnant Suicides	
Age	*Number*	*Percent*	*Number*	*Percent*
15–19	0	0	3	7
20–24	1	5	15	14
25–29	1	6	37	18
30–34	2	20	47	21
35–39	2	18	85	28
40–44	0	0	80	23
45–49	0	0	114	28

was transferred to a psychiatric hospital. There it was considered she was not mentally ill but, it was said, she had the usual problems arising from an unwanted pregnancy. She was allowed to discharge herself, and the social worker discussed organizations for unmarried mothers.

Mrs. B.M., aged 33, was 28 weeks pregnant when she died of barbiturate overdose. Her elder child, conceived when she was a prostitute, was adopted; the younger one, aged 5 and believed by the woman's future husband to be his, lived with relatives in Ireland. During the second pregnancy she attempted suicide by overdose. The birth was complicated and followed by a puerperal depression which required her first admission to a psychiatric hospital. Her husband had found her a burden then, and he was displeased about her being pregnant again; he demanded that either she move out or he would. She had been a patient in the psychiatric hospital for 11 weeks before her death and was home for weekend leave. She went out on her own, returned in the middle of the night, gathered together all her underclothing and set fire to the bundle. The next afternoon she told her husband she was going to confession. He found her dead in the bathroom at 11 PM. The several psychiatrists who had seen her thought she was a dullard who became depressed under stress, but an underlying schizophrenia was latterly suspected.

Miss B.U., aged 39, was 34 weeks pregnant when she drowned herself. She was previously healthy. For most of the time since her pregnancy had been medically confirmed, she was in an agitated depression and in a psychiatric hospital. The putative father was prepared to do the honorable thing, but he was unenthusiastic and she was undecided. Twice the wedding was arranged, and twice she refused to go to church. "I couldn't face the Priest like this" she explained the second time. Another wedding day was fixed, and the hospital resolved to keep her until the day and then escort her to church. However, she insisted on discharging herself two days before, and legally they could not stop her. Ten days later she was dead, but still not married.

Mrs. B.W. was 39, nulliparous, and five months pregnant when she drowned herself. Following a miscarriage, she had been subject to fits of depression for 12 months. They had become worse since she became pregnant again. She had had three admissions to a psychiatric hospital, and she had been admitted to a general hospital following a barbiturate overdose. She had returned home two weeks before her death, feeling much better after a week in hospital.

Mrs. C.O., aged 32, was 35 weeks pregnant when she gassed herself. She had been pleased to be pregnant although anxious in case she aborted, having had a spontaneous three-month abortion 12 months before. Then for a few weeks she had become increasingly depressed and worried about having a complicated labor. She had barely been two days in the psychiatric hospital when she went home and killed herself.

Mrs. C.L. was 29, married with three children, and three months pregnant when she took an overdose of a chloral and bromide sleeping mixture. For the past three and a half years she had been under almost continuous psychiatric care because of bouts of phobic depression. She had had five admissions to a psychiatric hospital during the period and was given modified insulin therapy, three long courses of electric convulsive therapy, and psychotherapy. She had attempted suicide with aspirin and twice with barbiturates. Her very experienced psychiatrist wrote to me: "I have no doubt that the pregnancy played a big part in the events leading to her death. A therapeutic termination was discussed but was not persisted with in any way, as she was very anxious to have the child."

EXTRAMARITALLY CONCEIVED PREGNANCIES AND EXPECTED ILLEGITIMATE BIRTHS

Of the 65 pregnancies, 40 or 61.5% had been extramaritally conceived (Table 5-3). There are no figures available to allow a comparison with all pregnancies in London AC. The percentage of all maternities in England and Wales conceived extramaritally was 12.7%. This is calculated from estimates for the same period which are provided in the registrar general's statistical reviews. It is only given for a rough guide: pregnancies aborted would have to be taken into consideration and so would the higher illegitimate rate in London AC.

Two of the women married after becoming pregnant, and it is reasonable to assume that there would have been more of them married before their babies were born if they had not killed themselves. For 27 of them, however, such a marriage would have been infeasible or unlikely. Eight were already married, but not to the putative father. Of these, seven were separated from their husbands.

Mrs. A.T. It is not certain that Mrs. A.T. was married. She told a nursing colleague that she was and that she had left her husband in

Table 5-3
Quinquennial Totals of Pregnant Suicides, Female Suicides (15–49), Total Live Births, and Illegitimate Births in London AC

Inclusive Years	Pregnant Suicides	Female Suicides Aged 15–49	Live Births in 1000s	Illegitimate Births in 1000s
1943–1947	13	345	274	23
1948–1952	7	359	275	15
1953–1957	14	425	256	20
1958–1962	31	567	289	34

Australia when she came to train in a London hospital, but she was known as Miss A.T. at the hospital. She became pregnant as a result of a sexual encounter at a party. All plans to return to Australia had been made and she did not want to return pregnant. She killed herself when she misunderstood her doctor and thought he was not going to recommend termination.

Mrs. A.Z. The husband of Mrs. A.Z. was a prisoner of war in Germany. From the note she left for the putative father, it seems he had let her down: "Perhaps now it's too late for you to ever understand. It's funny really, believing you loved me. Perhaps I was the bigger fool. It's just showed that, no matter what, I loved you."

Mrs. B.G. had been separated from her husband for two years and seems to have become pregnant during a chance encounter on her summer holiday.

Mrs. B.N. left her husband and seven children in Natal two years before. The putative father kept clear of her from the time her doctor confirmed her worst fears—or so it seemed to Mrs. B.N.

Mrs. B.Q. had been cohabiting with the putative father for over two years and her husband was in southern Rhodesia.

Mrs. B.R. had been given a legal separation, with custody of her two children, seven years before, and she lived with her parents. There is no information about the putative father.

Mrs. B.S. had been separated for an unstated time and lived with the putative father.

Mrs. C.A. The eighth woman, Mrs. C.A., had eloped for two months with the putative father but had returned to her matrimonial home for nearly two months. She had conceived during the elopement. She remained infatuated and her husband went to see the other man, begging him not to break up two homes, but he was told: "Women are only playthings to me."

Seven had become pregnant to married men.

Miss A.G. suffered from unrequited love towards her employer, a married man, and the putative father. She was a Cypriot and her note to him was in Greek: "My Darling—I should like very much not to call you my darling, not because I have stopped loving you but you don't deserve to be called my darling because you are not worthy of it—you are a thief—who does not steal ornaments but a thief of the peace of mind."

Miss A.N. had been living with the putative father, a married man, for the last eight months. During this time he had been associating with other women. When he was in hospital for teeth extraction, and received a telegram from another woman wishing him well, she was angry. So he told the coroner's officer. Instead of meeting him at the hospital the next day, as they had planned, she had him come home on his own and find her dead.

Miss B.C. had known the putative father for three years. He intended to marry her after he obtained a divorce he said, but legal proceedings had not begun.

Miss B.D., a German refugee, had been living with the putative father, a married man, for three years. She had taken her two illegitimate children when she joined him and she had two more by him. The putative father told the coroner's officer: "I was trying to get another room to live apart from her for a time" because she was making her annoyance at being pregnant again felt. Her note to him ended "I think to get out of trouble for you and the world I go, my life as such is no more worth living for me. My mind is all upside down, and you are to be blamed for it. But please forgive me."

Mrs. B.E. was Danish and divorced. During her 10 months in England, she had become friendly with the putative father. They visited her mother in Denmark because they were planning marriage. On their return to London he made off, telling her he already had a wife and five children. So she informed her mother in a short note.

Mrs. B.V. Her husband had been unfaithful and her divorce had come through four months before she took a fatal overdose of barbiturates. She had stayed with her mother for a time, but they did not get on. A friend took pity on her and invited her to stay at her home. Then began an affair with the friend's husband. At autopsy her uterus, enlarged with a two months' pregnancy, had a butterfly contraceptive in situ.

Miss C.P. was the senior nursing official of a large hospital. The putative father of her pregnancy, six months advanced when she died, was the administrator of the hospital and a married man.

In those days divorce proceedings were lengthy and for these 15 women only the sudden death of the innocent spouses would have made marriage legally attainable. Even so, as may be seen above, there would have been further problems facing at least half of them. In four cases the pregnancy had reached term, or almost, and there was really no time left for marriage.

Miss A.C., the student nurse, was 37 weeks pregnant when she came to London to kill herself.

Mrs. B.K., a widow, was actually in labor when she gassed herself and her two children.

Miss C.F. was 38 weeks pregnant when she drowned herself.

Miss C.K. was almost full-term when she gassed herself.

In three cases, from the report of the coroner's officer's interview with the putative father, there seems to have been no likelihood of marriage before the birth of the child.

Miss A.Q. met the putative father when they were fellow passengers on a ship from Australia. They lived together disharmoniously for four months, but then he moved off. She made an attempt to gas herself and was admitted to hospital. She told them there that she and her boyfriend were incompatible. On discharge she tracked him down, told him she had attempted suicide and moved into his new accommodation. Then she promised to move to a place of her own, but she drowned herself next day. Her boyfriend spoke of their incompatibility to the coroner's officer.

Miss A.R. lived with the putative father for the last six months before she gassed herself. He was training to be a teacher. They were to get married eventually, he told the coroner's officer, but not until he had finished training. This was not till nine months' time.

Mrs. B.L., a widow with five children, found them too much at times and was upset when she thought she might be pregnant again. The putative father told the coroner's officer: "I noticed she was jumpy and nervy and I decided that I should see less of her in future." She entered hospital for a hysterectomy because of fibroids and was told that her Hogben pregnancy test was positive—she went home and gassed herself. "You wouldn't think they would make me go on with it," she wrote to the putative father, but she did not wait to find out.

In two cases the woman had been jilted by the putative father and had begun a relationship with another man.

Miss A.F. had met her cohabiter in Wales nearly four months before she gassed herself. She was already pregnant, but the putative father would have nothing to do with her. She and her new boyfriend, a long-distance lorry driver, came to London to make a new start. They were to be married the next week. However, she worried about their finances and living in the one room they had rented and especially how they would manage with the baby as well.

Miss A.J. was 10 weeks pregnant. Bill, the putative father, gave her up six weeks before she gassed herself. She then became friendly with Ben and aimed at an early marriage. But she quarreled with Ben. It was all in her note to her mother: "I have not told you before but I think I am expecting a baby. I believe I am nearly three months . . . . The baby is not Ben's but Bill's. I don't know if you can ever forgive me . . . I did not want to bring disgrace to you. That was one reason why I was going to marry Ben so quickly. I do love Ben but I'm afraid we will not be happy. I walked out of my job today. What with your unhappiness, my work going wrong and I quarreled with Ben, and the baby as well, I feel I cannot go on. So I am putting myself to sleep for ever . . . ."

Two women had been about to marry the putative father but then declined.

Miss C.D., on being told by her doctor that she was five months pregnant, accompanied the putative father to a town in the north of England to be married, but she did not like the look of the town or the company he kept and changed her mind. He was a prisoner in Wormwood Scrubs for breaking and entering when she drowned herself.

Miss B.U. was the woman who had three wedding ceremonies arranged but each time she could not bring herself to turn up.

Finally, there was one pregnant girl who was only 14 when she conceived.

Miss A.A. was 10 weeks pregnant when she gassed herself. The 18-year-old youth who was the putative father had continued to see her despite the growing disapproval of her parents. She did not confide in her mother because she was afraid of what her father would do to her lover. The immediate precipitant of her suicide was the prospect of a row in the morning with her father for coming in late. It seems clear that the father would not have consented to the marriage of this schoolgirl daughter.

For the remaining 11, the prospect of marriage might have been less bleak.

Miss C.E. For Miss C.E., aged 23, the prospect of marriage seems to have been good. She would not have known for sure that she was pregnant, for her pregnancy was only four weeks advanced. She did not express concern to her boyfriend, and she made no mention of pregnancy to her sister in whom she always confided. Her boyfriend had known her for five years, since before he joined the Fleet Air Arm. They had met five times in the six weeks since his return from abroad. When his leave finished, she saw him off at the railway station and then jumped in front of another train.

Miss A.U. Two men wanted to marry Miss A.U., a 25-year-old model, but she seems to have played one off against the other. She had been engaged to Tim, but broke off 13 weeks before her death to become engaged to Tom. She continued to see Tim. She told Tom she was going to model at a fashion show in Paris, and he was going to join her in a few days. She told Tim she was going to model in a fashion house in London. Tim was going to give her a lift there, but when he called he found her dead from coal-gas poisoning. It turned out that the Paris and London establishments had never heard of her.

Three had an illegitimate child already. With characters already stained, there might have been less pressure for a shotgun marriage.

Mrs. B.B., aged 27 and a widow for seven years, lived with the putative father. Their 5-year-old daughter had recently been sent to a boarding school. His marital status is not recorded, but perhaps he was already married.

Miss A.K., four months pregnant, had been keeping company with a divorced man for two years. Her child was adopted when she met him. For four weeks she had been living with him. This was to save money for the baby, he said. He made no reference to marriage plans, although he mentioned her abortion attempts.

Miss A.H., aged 20, was a drop-out and would not have been too concerned about social conventions. The baby she had when she was 16 was adopted. She had been living with her current boyfriend for nine weeks, which was the length of her pregnancy. In a state of collapse, she told him at one o'clock in the morning that she had taken an overdose of her hayfever tablets. She died two hours later of diphenhydramine poisoning. Apparently she did not tell him she was pregnant.

In the remaining six cases there is no information about the putative father.

Miss A.B. was 18 when she swallowed 300 aspirin tablets. She was sick, and she told her mother she had taken them because she was pregnant. While her mother fetched the doctor, she told her father she had tried many abortifacients, but she refused to name the putative father.

Miss A.V., 25, and four weeks pregnant, also lived at home. Her mother knew she had been worrying about her period not appearing, but she did not know she had a boyfriend.

Miss A.Y., 26, and eight weeks pregnant, shared a flat with another girl. Neither her flatmate nor her father knew of a boyfriend. Neither boyfriend nor pregnancy is mentioned in the note she left for a girlfriend: "My darling, when you get this I shall be dead. I can't go on any longer—no good at anything or to anybody. If there is a hell, I might as well get there sooner or later—what's a few years extra in eternity? I can only pray that my evil has not tainted you in any way, because you were my friend, in the very truest sense. May God bless you always."

Miss B.J., 31, lived at home, but her parents did not know she was nine weeks pregnant or had a boyfriend. They did not even know she had not been to work the two previous days, until after she jumped in front of a train and a letter was found from her employer asking for an explanation of her absence.

Miss B.Z., 39, and 13 weeks pregnant, lived on her own. She had obtained from her doctor a hormone pregnancy test without discussing the circumstances of the suspected pregnancy. There was no family to question for she had come from Russia via a displaced persons' camp in Germany 13 years before.

Miss C.M., aged 31, also lived on her own. She had already taken an overdose of aspirin—when she was four weeks pregnant. She had been feeling sick, but there was an inquiry about why she was not at work. This was her reason for taking them. Twenty-four weeks later, on the night of her death from barbiturate overdose, a man phoned the local police to say: "Miss C.M. phoned me to say goodbye as she had taken poison, so I called you up." But he was not interviewed by the coroner's officer. There is no more information about him or their relationship.

In short, if all the 65 women had gone on to have their babies instead of killing themselves, between 27 and 38 would have been illegitimate—that is to say 42% to 58%. This is five to seven times the illegitimate rate in London AC during the period. The apparent relationship between suicide during pregnancy and illegitimacy also appears in the fall and rise of both during the 20 years studied, as may be seen in Table 5-3.

STAGE OF PREGNANCY

Those women with extramaritally conceived pregnancies tended to kill themselves in the earlier months of pregnancy; this is demonstrated in Table 5-4.

The stage of pregnancy that the women had reached when they committed suicide ranged from the first month to labor; this is shown in Table 5-5. There was a big peak during the third month and a small one during the last month. The women in these two groups were of the same age distribution, but there was a larger proportion of women with extramaritally conceived pregnancies among those who killed themselves during the third month of their pregnancy. They amounted to 14 of 17 (82%).

They have been mentioned in the previous section:

Miss A.A., Miss A.B., Miss A.G., Miss A.H., Miss A.J., Miss A.R., Mrs. A.Z., Mrs. B.B., Miss B.D., Miss B.J., Mrs. B.L., Mrs. B.S., Mrs. B.V., and Mrs. C.A.

Of the three who were married, two had intolerable marriages.

Mrs. A.D. was 19 and 10 weeks pregnant. She had a shotgun marriage when she was 16. Her husband had been giving her beatings for at least two years—since she was pregnant with her second child which he continued to maintain was not his. Her sister described some of the beatings she had witnessed and tried to stop. He was disputing the paternity of her third pregnancy, and she ran away for a week. She returned to London and told her sister she was going to risk a beating to see her children, who were by then with her mother-in-law. On reaching her empty home, she wrote a letter to her sister and in the middle of it she decided to take her life. "I have left James by now, you should know. I have got no

Table 5-4
Marital Status and Duration of Pregnancy

Marital State at Time of Conception	Duration of Pregnancy at Time of Suicide (weeks)	
	4–16	*17–40*
Living in wedlock	5	20
Living out of wedlock*	25	15

*Unmarried, separated, widowed, divorced.

Table 5-5
Number of Women in Each Four Weeks of Pregnancy at Time of Suicide

Duration of Pregnancy at Time of Suicide			
Weeks	*Number*	*Weeks*	*Number*
4	2	21–24	6
5– 8	3	25–28	5
9–12	17	29–32	3
13–16	8	33–36	2
17–20	9	37–40	10

money and I need some but I have not got an address yet so when I do would you please write to me and let me know how Winnie and David are getting on. Would you please tell James there is no other man? I left him because of his temper and my nerves are dead now. If only he did not treat me like he did I would still be with him. I have not had anything to eat for three days now and I am very hungry. I have got a girl friend with me and she is in the same boat as I am—you know what I mean. I love the children very much and I love James too but he treated me like a pig and I could not stand it any more. Please do not think I am a bad girl because I have not done anything wrong. I know James will kill me when he sees me but there won't be any need for it as I might do it myself. My father was not frightened and I am not. Anyhow I will be with mummy won't I? Your loving sister." When her husband came home from work he found her in the kitchen lying on a blanket with her head on a pillow on the open door of the gas oven, fully clothed and dead.

Mrs. B.X. was 39 and had six children. The eldest two, who were by a previous marriage, had left home as soon as an opportunity presented itself. Mr. B.X. was inclined to come home drunk from work and be violent towards his wife and four children, so his eldest child, a daughter aged 13, told the coroner's officer. Mrs. B.X. had been ill in bed with bronchitis the day before her death. When her husband came home at ten o'clock there was no meal ready for him. His daughter was dispatched for jellied eels. By the time she returned, her father was hitting her mother with his belt. Mrs. B.X. ran out of the house and later returned with a policeman, but by this time Mr. B.X. had gone to bed. Mrs. B.X. spent the night in the kitchen. In the morning before Mr. B.X. went off to work there was another row: Mrs. B.X. had taken five shillings of the rent money to buy an abortifacient. Later in the morning she sent a daughter to their doctor for a prescription for amylobarbitone sodium. The doctor said she took on average 1 gram a day and was thereby "able to maintain a fairly normal life and do her best to look after her family." As she was dropping into her last sleep, she told her son, aged 9: "I've taken a drug. I've always loved you all."

The seventeenth, in striking contrast, enjoyed a happy marriage and looked forward to having her baby. From the available information, an early schizophrenia best accounts for her death.

Mrs. C.H., 10 weeks pregnant, was happy to be pregnant again. In the few weeks before her death, her doctor told me a year later, she seemed happier than at any time he had known her. During this time she had become confirmed into the Church of England. Her only problem during her pregnancy was insomnia, and she was prescribed barbiturates. Her elder daughter, aged 7, came home from school and found her mother unconscious with a white prayer book in one hand, a white handkerchief in the other, and a white box on the floor. A few hours later she had died from barbiturate poisoning.

Of the 10 women who went through to the last month of pregnancy, only four had extramaritally conceived pregnancies, that is to say 40%. From the available evidence they told no one, and it occurred to no one, that they were pregnant. They were of cheerful disposition, according to the records, and showed no evidence of anxiety. It was as if they concealed the fact of their pregnancies from everyone including themselves, cheerfully going on as if nothing unusual was happening.

Miss A.C. was the student nurse who came to London to kill herself. No one at her hospital seemed to have had any idea that she was pregnant. It appears that the senior nursing official did not know until I was making inquiries six years later. Miss A.C. did not consult her doctor. She lost no time from her duties and appeared perfectly fit until the day she gassed herself. "She was a pleasant happy girl. She did not appear moody, as if worried."

Miss C.F. lived at home with the rest of the family, but apparently they did not know she was pregnant. Occasionally she was in the company of Mr. P.Q., but on her death he denied having had sexual relations with her. He knew that she had met a boyfriend during her summer holiday. She had consulted her doctor about a vaginal discharge when her pregnancy was five months advanced, and he prescribed a medicine for her to take. Her mother said she had a happy, jolly disposition and was on good terms with everybody. She had never given her mother any cause for anxiety in the past. She was not courting, and she had had no love affairs.

Miss C.K. Her boyfriend visited her in her furnished rooms every day. He told the coroner's officer he had noticed she had put on weight in recent months, but he did not know she was pregnant. He did admit having had sexual intercourse with her. Her medical notes had been destroyed by the time I inquired, but her doctor recalled how she had come to have her pregnancy confirmed and how she had shown no resentment. He was struck with her tranquillity. Her boyfriend said she was a cheerful and happy girl.

Mrs. B.K. Her sister-in-law said she and her daughter both noticed that Mrs. B.K. was getting stout, but they did not have the slightest idea that she was pregnant. This fits in with a note she left for her sister-in-law. "My dear sister, dare I ask you for forgiveness for the tragedy I am causing you, as, apart from the children, you are all I have in the world, but I am so ashamed of myself I could not bring myself to face you and tell you I am pregnant. You and Jill may have noticed but said nothing, for which I am grateful. I am taking the children with me although God knows it breaks my heart. But if I leave them who will look after them—no one, and apart from that I couldn't bear them answering in later life the consequences of my ill-doing. I have been in terrible agony the past three days and nights mentally and physically as I have had a show, losing clots of blood, and the pain I can't bear any longer . . . . So goodbye and God bless you. P.S. Do not try to find out who the father is of my unborn child as it won't pay you to but anyway it is exactly nine months." There was no reference to her being of cheerful disposition but she was obviously thoughtful and generous, and it is compatible.

As for the quality of the six marriages, it varied, but it was never like that of the two atrocious marriages mentioned above.

Mrs. C.G. normally had a good relationship with her husband. On the Sunday night of her death, he had gone out with his brother, and they did not return till the early hours. She began to give him a tongue-lashing for this, but he cut her short by walking into the bedroom. She poured a can of paraffin over herself, lit a piece of paper from the stove, and put it to her coat. As she did so she burst into flames.

Mrs. A.W. Her husband had been in hospital for the past three months, and she was meanwhile living with her brother. The latter said she was looking forward to having the baby, but not to the birth. On the day of her death, she had been told at the antenatal clinic that she would have to go to hospital for the birth. She had made all the preparations to have the baby at home.

Mrs. C.J. was looking forward to having her baby. However, she had become anxious and depressed, fearful that she was going to die, and she was admitted to hospital 10 days before the delivery was expected. Her solicitous husband was also anxious. She left the ward saying that she was going to have a wash, broke the cabinet for the fire-escape key, and climbed on to a parapet. As a doctor approached, she stepped off and fell to her death.

Mrs. B.A. and her husband had had arguments about the paternity of the pregnancy. He alleged she had been associating with another man. There was a row over this when she was four months pregnant, and she had tried to gas herself. After that he did not mention the matter. On the night of her death she appeared quite normal, put her two children to bed, but gassed herself instead of following her husband to bed.

Mrs. B.P. had poor eyesight since childhood, and it had recently deteriorated further. Six weeks before her death, she had an operation for a detached retina, and she feared there had not been any improvement. She had been looking forward to having a second baby, but lately she felt she would not be able to cope. Before she gassed herself, she wrote a note to her husband: "Not much time to write, please understand this is the only way out of a very bad dilemma which can only lead to much worse. All love."

Mrs. C.B. was living with her husband, although she was promiscuous and had lived with other men before and since marriage. Four of her six children were by her husband. She had vomited off and on throughout the pregnancy. It was unwanted, as she made clear to the doctors two weeks before when she was admitted to hospital for a week on account of backache. She had attempted to gas herself two years before when living with another man. This time she took an overdose of barbiturates. She left a note for her husband: "My darling Bill, if anything happens to me it is because of this terrible pain in my back. I can't go on. It's too much. Sorry I couldn't hang on any longer, love. Thank you for everything. Try not to think hard of me. I couldn't stand it any longer. I hope you will never suffer it. God bless you. Your loving wife."

PARITY

It appears from the records that there were 38 nulliparae, but in a few cases it is possible that the woman was parous without the coroner's officer being able to ascertain it. The excess of nulliparous over parous women was among middle-trimester suicides. Eleven of the women had one child; eight had two; two had three; two had four; one had five; two had six; and one had seven. Of the four grand multiparae, two were living in wedlock, one was separated, and one widowed.

Ten of the parous women, because of various circumstances, did not have their children living with them.

Miss A.H. and **Miss A.K.** both had their children adopted.

Mrs. B.B. had recently sent her 5-year-old illegitimate daughter to boarding school. Both her father and her cohabiter said she had been depressed since then.

Mrs. B.M. Her elder child was adopted and her younger child stayed with relatives in Ireland.

Mrs. B.S. had recently returned upset from visiting her war-evacuated 11-year-old son and had unsuccessfully sought his transfer to another billet.

Mrs. B.N. Her seven children were in Natal. She had not saved sufficient money during her two years as a hospital orderly to bring them to London.

Mrs. B.P. Her 2½-year-old daughter stayed with her grandparents, probably because of Mrs. B.P.'s failing eyesight.

Mrs. B.Q. Her son, like his father, lived in southern Rhodesia.

Mrs. B.V., divorced and without a home of her own, did not have her son living with her.

Mrs. C.A. Her son was 19 and serving overseas in the Royal Navy.

Thus only 17 of the 65 had a child or children living with them.

THE DUAL EFFECT OF PREGNANCY

Pregnancy works both ways. It may influence a woman toward suicide, and it may protect her from it. Pregnancy is part of the basic biological process which perpetuates the human race. This may not be exactly in the forefront of a woman's mind if she is having months of unrelieved nausea or if she has landed in a desperate social plight, but she will have some sort of primitive need within her to protect the growing fetus.

Example 39-year-old Miss B.U. struggled, until her pregnancy was 34 weeks advanced, with the dilemma between the ignominy of having an illegitimate child and entering a loveless shotgun marriage. As she jumped feet first into the canal, she was heard to cry: "Oh my baby!"

It also works both ways in a population. There were a few women, as will have been noted, who killed themselves because they were pregnant. There were also a few who wanted to be pregnant and killed themselves because they were not.

Example Four women killed themselves because they feared they could not bear a child, according to the records. Three were married and living with their husbands, two were aged 30 and one was 38. One was married and separated. She feared her cohabiter would leave her because she seemed unable to have children. She was 31.

In some cases the social or physical effect of the pregnancy was apparently the last straw and in others a contributory factor towards suicide; at the other end of the scale, it is reasonable to assume, becoming pregnant alone prevented some women from killing themselves and was a contributory factor for others surviving.

The protective effect of pregnancy might be expected to be stronger and the suicide effect weaker in women over 25 than in women under 25, for women over 25 are more likely to be married and wanting to have children or at least prepared to have them. This accords with Table 5-6, a rough comparison of the incidence of pregnancy among female suicides (Suicides in London AC) with the incidence of pregnancy in the general population (London AC min/max). It is rough because there are no age-related figures regarding women in London AC, so those for greater London have been used. London AC is the central part of greater London,

Table 5-6
Estimated Incidences* of Macroscopically Discernible Pregnancy among Female Suicides in London AC and in the General Population of London AC

	Women aged 15–24		Women aged 25–34		Women aged 35–44	
Inclusive Years	*London AC min–max*†	*Suicides in London AC*	*London AC min–max*†	*Suicides in London AC*	*London AC min–max*†	*Suicides in London AC*
1948–1952	40–45	67	61–68	42	17–19	13
1953–1957	45–50	156	61–68	42	14–16	13
1958–1962	57–63	183	71–78	64	16–18	33

*Incidence of frequency per 1000.
†The minimum and maximum estimations for women in greater London were derived from Tables of Estimated Populations by Sex and Age and Tables of Total Numbers of Maternities According to Age of Mother in the Registrar General's Statistical Review of England and Wales for the years 1948 to 1962. The figures for greater London were then adjusted to accommodate London AC's lower birth rate. These tables were not supplied in the reviews for the years 1943–1947 (being war years and intermediate post-war years. The review comes out annually). The following assumptions were made in the estimations: (1) pregnancies were macroscopically discernible at four weeks and thereafter; (2) the rate of spontaneous and induced abortion at any age group of mothers was between 10 and 40% of all pregnancies; (3) the mean duration of gestation was between 39 and 41 weeks; and (4) the mean duration of pregnancies ending in abortion of any kind was between 8 and 11.5 weeks.

and its population is 40% of the whole. Life in the middle of a conurbation is different from life in its suburbs. The birth rate of London AC was lower, and the figures have been adjusted for this. But there are many other differences.

It can be seen that, among the young women, a suicide was more likely to be pregnant than a nonsuicide woman—and increasingly so during the 15-year period for which figures are available. On the other hand, among women in the older groups, a suicide was less likely to be pregnant during the first two quinquennia, although in the last quinquennium the suicides in the oldest group had caught up so that, as in the youngest group, pregnancy increased the suicide risk.

INDUCED ABORTION

In considering the individual cases, there is often striking evidence of pregnancy motivating the woman towards suicide. Although certain items have been extracted above—suicide was more likely to occur in young single women without prospect of marrying the putative father, without children, and in their third month of pregnancy—most of the evidence eludes statistical presentation. There were some women in which it seems to have exerted little or no influence, but in many cases the social effect of the pregnancy seems to have been largely responsible for the suicide, and in a few there is strong direct evidence (in the form of suicide note or death-bed statement, for instance) that the pregnancy was the immediate precipitating factor. One case shades into another.

In light of this, we might expect many of the women to have been rejected abortion applicants. It would certainly have been expected to be so at the time. During the last seven years of the period, 122 abortions were performed in the Samaritan Hospital, the gynecology department of St. Mary's Hospital, London. Forty-nine were performed because of physical illnesses, 17 because of maternal rubella, and the remaining 56 because of psychiatric reasons. Forty of the psychiatric recommendations were available for my inspection, and 23 of them alluded to suicidal risk. What happened to those women whose request for therapeutic abortion was denied?

Surprisingly, from the available evidence, none of the 65 pregnant suicides had sought a termination of pregnancy and been refused. One woman killed herself, perhaps more in pique than in despair, when she thought her doctor was stringing her along; one woman who was in hospital waiting to see the gynecologist about her newly confirmed, and unwanted, pregnancy went home and gassed herself; and in two cases a psychiatric recommendation for therapeutic abortion would have been made but the women did not want it. These four women have been mentioned already in some detail.

Mrs. A.T., aged 24, was returning to Australia in seven weeks' time. Her doctor knew her well, for throughout her nursing training he supported her through bouts of depression. She was also troubled with menstrual irregularity. She consulted him because her period was exceptionally late and she had had intercourse on one occasion at a party. The pregnancy test was negative. She returned because her period still had not arrived. He could not examine her satisfactorily because of vaginismus, but the second pregnancy test was negative. On her next visit, it was all too easy to feel her enlarged uterus abdominally. He tried hard to reassure her, and he had in mind asking a gynecologist if he would terminate the pregnancy, even though it was by now 20 weeks advanced. She became extremely hostile, presumably believing he had deliberately led her on. "There is only one thing to do," she snapped. She was implacable and ran off. She had just moved and had not given him her new address. He was unable to trace her through her friends. Long before, she had told him that she had accumulated a fatal quantity of barbiturates in case life ever became too much for her, and it had been this that she had taken.

Mrs. B.L., aged 33 and a widow with five children aged 9–15, feared she might be pregnant when she came into hospital for a hysterectomy because of fibroids and a Hogben test confirmed her fears. The putative father had arranged to visit the hospital, but he decided it was time to cool the relationship. She wrote to him. "I promised to write to you after my op. Well, as I thought, I can't have it because I am pregnant. I don't know what to do now. There's no going back, and I can't face going on. You wouldn't think they would make me go on with it. It will only make matters a hundred times worse than they are already. I haven't had any visitors and I shan't get any now, but I have got my case here so that I can go home without worrying anyone." She must have gone home immediately after writing this, an hour before she was due to be interviewed by the gynecologist, and gassed herself.

Mrs. C.L., aged 29, married to a busy professional man, with three children aged 5, 4, and 1, was three months pregnant. For the past three and a half years she had been having attacks of depression, insomnia, fatigue, anorexia, phobias, and ruminations about insanity and disease. She had had a great deal of psychiatric treatment. For the past six weeks she had suffered frequent nausea and was in bed most of the time. Three years before she had had a therapeutic abortion. She expressed some guilt to her psychiatrist at the time, but it improved her condition and she did not express any further guilt. Another therapeutic abortion was suggested, for her psychiatrist felt it would have helped in her final illness, but she declined.

Mrs. B.M. The first psychiatrist who saw Mrs. B.M. in her final illness observed that she was very depressed and had recently taken an overdose. He also noted that she had made a suicide attempt during the depression she had in her other pregnancy. But he went on to record: "There is absolutely no desire on her part to have a termination of her pregnancy as she wants the child and is very fond of children."

Perhaps more of the women would have sought a therapeutic abortion, if it had been as easily available as it is nowadays; there are now some 30 times as many performed at the Samaritan Hospital as there were during the seven years quoted above, for example. However, the number would still have been minute in terms of London AC over 20 years. It was to self-abortion and to criminal abortion that women turned with unwanted pregnancies. There is no way of knowing their numbers, but the coroners' depositions have evidence of fatalities arising when these operations went wrong. Two hundred seventy-six deaths arising from abortion were recorded by the London coroners during 1943–1962, the number falling greatly in the second decade presumably because of the introduction of antibiotics. Of these, 90 were found to have been caused by the woman herself, 75 by other persons known or unknown, and 111 were left "open" or undetermined by the coroners.

CHAPTER 6

PREGNANCY, SUICIDE, AND ATTEMPTED SUICIDE: Marital Status, Interpersonal Relations, and Social Factors

F.A. WHITLOCK

Children are the anchors that hold a mother to life

Phaedra, Sophocles

Despite the enormous number of papers and books reporting epidemiological, psychological, and forensic aspects of suicide and attempted suicide, very few comment in any detail on the number of suicide victims found to be pregnant at the time. Similarly, few authors report on the frequency of suicidal behavior during pregnancy. A number of official surveys of maternal mortality pay some attention to this issue, but on examination of these investigations, it is clear that the majority of suicides associated with pregnancy occur during the puerperium. This is not to say that suicide during pregnancy never occurs, but there is no contemporary evidence documenting a high incidence of suicidal deaths in the course of gestation.

On the other hand, time and place may well be important factors in pregnancy-associated suicide rates. McClure et al (1971), for example, have quoted figures dating from 1900 to 1962, mainly from countries in continental Europe, claiming that some 13.5% of women between the ages of 12 and 50 who committed suicide were pregnant when they took their lives. Their figures tell us very little but, assuming that a large percentage of these victims were single or carrying an extranuptial pregnancy, it is not difficult to imagine that public attitudes in earlier times might have been powerful determinants of the suicidal act. Today, at least in many Western countries, less shame, fortunately, is attached to these situations and, one might conjecture, the pressure on the woman to take her life might well have lessened. In addition, greater facilities for abortion have provided an alternative to suicide when an unwanted pregnancy has been conceived. To what extent some self-induced or "backyard" abortions in the past could be interpreted as suicidal acts by women who felt themselves to be in desperate, irremediable situations cannot be estimated.

SUICIDES IN PREGNANCY

Most commentators have declared that suicide during pregnancy is an infrequent event. Just how infrequent is demonstrated by mortality data during pregnancy from Australia between 1964 and 1975 (Maternal Deaths in the Commonwealth of Australia, 1964–1975) and England and Wales between 1967 and 1975 (Reports on Confidential Enquiries into Maternal Deaths in England and Wales, 1967–1975). In Australia, there were 2,890,389 confinements, during which 26 mothers died by suicide or "accidents," giving an overall rate of 0.9 per 100,000 confinements. In England and Wales, there were 6,677,211 maternities, 17 of which ended in suicide, a rate of 0.5 per 100,000. These figures are far below the "normal" suicide rates for those aged 15–45, and are comparable with Barno's (1967) figure of 0.3 per 100,000 pregnancies in Minnesota between 1950 and 1965. The question arises, why did these women take their lives?

In Barno's series, all four women were in the last weeks of pregnancy, and all were diagnosed as suffering from psychotic depression. It appears, therefore, that severe mental illness was the main cause of suicide, as it so often is in patients who take their lives during the puerperium, often within a few weeks of delivery.

In England and Wales less is known about the precise mental states of the 17 victims. One case was a single girl who took her life after 10 weeks of pregnancy. Another was a Pakistani woman who spoke no English, who died at 28 weeks. A third was four months pregnant but had been refused abortion and took an overdose of chloral. A fourth victim had also asked for an abortion. Another multiparous, married woman tried to abort herself, failed, and then took her life. A 16-year-old girl was eight weeks pregnant when she committed suicide, and one woman asked for termination at 34 weeks but died from an overdose of barbiturates.

Even less is known about the Australian victims, but eight suicides occurred early in pregnancy and one late. The majority of deaths resulted from overdoses of barbiturates or carbon monoxide poisoning. It was assumed that those who killed themselves early in pregnancy were severely depressed at the time, and a number of puerperal suicides occurred in women with past histories of psychiatric disorders. Goodwin and Harris (1979) reported their findings on three women who committed suicide at 14, 26, and 37 weeks, respectively. All were married, and the suicidal acts followed major altercations with their husbands. To what extent the pregnancies contributed to emotional instability sufficient to cause suicide is not discussed, as the authors were more concerned to draw an analogy between these women's deaths and that of Hedda Gabler in Ibsen's drama, who shot herself when finding herself pregnant rather than accept her feminine role as a mother.

It is impossible to draw any general conclusions from these reports which provide insufficient data on the victims' mental states before they died. No particular period of pregnancy seems more conducive to suicide than any other, but all of Barno's cases were in the last weeks of pregnancy. One might conjecture that suicide late in pregnancy is more likely to be associated with severe depression or psychosis, whereas suicide in the early weeks might be interpreted as a reaction to a situation seen by the victim as beyond remedy. One cannot assume that the pregnancy alone was the sole cause of these suicides, as a host of psychosocial variables might have contributed. As McMurdo has pointed out, leaving aside frank psychotic illnesses, single status, financial difficulty, and loss of support by the putative father as well as rejection by the girl's family could tip the balance toward death which would not have occurred had circumstances been more favorable.

If one turns to surveys of cohorts of suicide, again the information is often insufficient. In an investigation of 1052 suicides in England and Wales, based on coroners' reports, there were 127 women aged 15–44 (Whitlock, 1977). Two of these women were pregnant at the time and a third, a single girl, falsely believed she was pregnant and took her life after a dispute with her boyfriend. Both the other women were married and died within the first few months of pregnancy. In one case there was much marital discord, and the husband was said to be morbidly jealous. In the other, there was a history of previous suicide attempts and numerous miscarriages which had been a major source of worry to the patient. Thus, the suicide rate in this group of women was 1.57%. Against this figure, one finds Otto (1965) quoting an incidence of pregnancy in women who had committed suicide ranging from 3% to 20%, figures based mainly on continental European reports. Taylor et al (1964) in South London reported on 100 female suicides, of whom approximately 20 would have been beyond the childbearing age. There were three pregnant suicides, giving an incidence of 3.5%. No details for the reasons for these women taking their lives are available beyond the fact that one patient suicided shortly after a self-induced threatened abortion. Seager and Flood (1965) investigated 136 female deaths by suicide in Bristol, of whom 43 were aged less than 50. There were three cases of pregnancy in this group, giving an incidence of 7%. Potondi (1965) in Budapest found that 1.1% of 1000 female suicides were pregnant. Presumably this included all age groups, and the rate would have been higher had the report been restricted to those of childbearing age.

Taking these reports together, it does appear that between 1% and 7% of women aged 15–45 who take their lives are pregnant at the time. Unfortunately, we have only meager information about the reasons for their actions, but one has the impression that in only a small number of cases is the pregnancy the sole or even the major cause.

Histories of previous suicide attempts, grave marital disturbances, and other psychosocial factors may compound with the pregnancy to produce a situation where feelings of desperation may be sufficient to tilt the balance to death rather than to life. One might surmise that those who died during the first trimester were less likely to be suffering from major mental illnesses than those who took their lives in the terminal months of the pregnancy. It has been argued that with the onset of quickening, the mother becomes more aware of and concerned for the safety of the infant she will bear. The knowledge that taking her own life would also cause the death of the fetus might well be sufficient to deter the potential suicide victim from proceeding further with any plans for action. The element of speculation in these comments must be acknowledged but, in truth, we know far too little about what determines or prevents suicide during pregnancy. Certainly, it is an uncommon event, but it remains one which would justify further investigation.

ATTEMPTED SUICIDES

In contrast to actual suicide, suicidal behavior classed as attempted suicide is not uncommon. Whitlock and Edwards (1968) reported on 30 suicide attempts in women aged less than 45 who were contrasted with 369 nonpregnant women of the same age group. Ten of the pregnant patients were aged less than 20, and 18 were between 20 and 29. Although there were rather more single women than in the general population, it was not a statistically significant finding. On the other hand, the six women who were divorced or separated were in excess of the expected number based on whole population figures. The frequency of attempted suicide in the pregnant group was 7.5% of the whole cohort, a figure no different from the expected number of pregnant women in the community (7%) at any given time. Eleven of the pregnant women (36.5%) had received psychiatric treatment in the past, a figure which was no different from the 38% in the nonpregnant patients. Two pregnant women were manifestly suffering from major psychiatric illnesses, schizophrenia in one case and endogenous depression in another. On follow-up 12–18 months later, it is noteworthy that none of the pregnant women had died by suicide, whereas this had been the cause of death in seven of the nonpregnant patients.

Bearing in mind that the suicide attempt was often triggered by a violent dispute, inquiry was made into the quality of the relationship between the patient and her husband or lover. In seven cases these relationships were described as good or satisfactory, in two it was impossible to say definitely what circumstances prevailed at the time of the suicide attempt, but for the remaining 21 patients the relationship was thoroughly unsatisfactory. Desertion or threats of desertion were frequent, and the marital relationships were marred by recurrent rows. The actual adjustment of the patients was good in seven cases, bad in 12, and unknown in 11. In summary, therefore, it can be said with some confidence that this sample of women had a marked incapacity for stable human and sexual relationships. The contribution made by this factor to the ultimate suicide attempt was probably greater than the pregnancy itself.

For 16 patients this was their first pregnancy and for five, their second. The remaining nine patients had two or more earlier pregnancies, not necessarily resulting in live births, and one patient had borne six children before the present pregnancy.

The suicide attempt took place during the first trimester in 14 patients, in the second in 13, in the last trimester for the remaining three cases. Seventeen of the mothers wanted to have their babies and 13 definitely did not. The child had been conceived in wedlock by 14 of the women, premaritally by 12, extramaritally by four. It was considered that in five patients the pregnancy was the principal cause of the suicide attempt, a partial cause in eight patients, and more or less irrelevant or incidental in the remaining 17. These judgments imply that as far as the first group is concerned, the suicide attempt would not have occurred had the patient not been pregnant, whereas for the second group the pregnancy was a contributory cause. However, it was felt that with 17 patients the suicide attempt was unconnected with the pregnancy, although it is impossible to rule out some temporary emotional instability or stress caused by the pregnancy, so contributing to an impulsive suicidal attempt often precipitated by a major dispute.

The following are examples of some of the patients illustrating the nature of the suicide attempts and the circumstances in which they took place.

Case 1 A 16-year-old shop assistant took a handful of aspirin impulsively after a row with her boyfriend who had refused to take her to a party. He was not responsible for the patient's pregnancy, now in its 16th week, and there was no evidence that the pregnancy was the cause of the suicide attempt. The patient was regarded as an unstable immature personality whose behavior had been precipitated by a brief interpersonal crisis. The father of the child had deserted her. Ultimately the baby was born normally and adopted, but when the patient was seen eight months later she was anxious and depressed, complaining of loss of interest and, perhaps justifiably, a fear of sex.

Case 2 The patient was an 18-year-old single shop assistant who made an impulsive suicide attempt with barbiturates, following a row with her mother who refused to allow her to marry. The patient came from a broken home and reacted violently to the circumstances of her life at the time. She was anxious to continue with the pregnancy, now of two months' duration. In the end she married and was reported to be alive and well 18 months after her suicide attempt. It was felt that, although the dispute with her mother had precipitated her action, the existence of the pregnancy also contributed to the situational crisis.

Case 3 A 28-year-old woman, married but separated from her husband, had a row with her de facto husband who was responsible for her pregnancy. As this man wished to leave her, she impulsively took a quantity of barbiturates with the expressed intention of dying. She showed features of a neurotic depressive reaction and a vulnerable, unstable personality. Her relationship with her lover was wholly unsatisfactory, but she was anxious to have her baby. Despite this, the baby was adopted. The pregnancy in this case did not contribute significantly to the suicidal attempt.

Case 4 A 17-year-old factory worker, three months pregnant, took an overdose of carbrital after a row with her fiancé one day before the wedding. The existence of the pregnancy probably contributed to the suicidal behavior. Ultimately, she married and the baby was born six months later. When seen one year after her suicide attempt, she was depressed and had made further suicide attempts during her second pregnancy. The marriage was very unhappy, and her husband was planning to leave her.

Case 5 A 26-year-old single woman, temporarily unemployed, impulsively slashed her wrists and took an overdose of barbiturates. She had made a similar suicide attempt some two years previously. Her present action was precipitated by her pregnancy, which was wanted, and by worry over her job. She came from a broken home, was addicted to barbiturates, and showed many of the features of sociopathic personality. Her relationship to the father of her child was very unsatisfactory, and she was sexually frigid. She was in the first trimester of her pregnancy. The baby was born normally, and she later married a man who was not the child's father. Six weeks after marriage she was admitted to hospital with a diagnosis of amphetamine psychosis. Two weeks later, following discharge, she was again admitted following a serious suicide attempt with barbiturates. The baby was later adopted, following the patient's admission to a mental hospital. Seven months later the patient was readmitted after a further suicide attempt. She was now four months pregnant and very unhappily married. She had thought of procuring an abortion but took no action in the matter. It was felt that the patient's second and fourth suicide attempts were in part caused by the pregnancies.

What is particularly noteworthy in this study is the lack of major differences between the pregnant and nonpregnant suicidal population. The pregnant women were slightly younger and, consequently, more often unmarried than the nonpregnant group, but these differences were of little significance. Other social factors did not separate these two groups. The pregnant women tended to be more impulsive in their behavior and made use of a rather wider selection of drugs in their suicide attempts. Nonetheless, both groups predominantly used barbiturates.

Interestingly, although similar proportions of the two groups were alone at the time of their suicidal act, significantly more of the pregnant women sought help afterwards. This may have been due to their greater immaturity or because so many of these women were in situations which consciously or unconsciously they hoped would be influenced by their behavior. In contrast to the nonpregnant patients, only one patient made a further suicide attempt during the ensuing months. This is explicable on the grounds that so many of the attempts were precipitated by short-lived acute crises which were unlikely to recur. Either the suicidal act "worked," in that it produced a change in the circumstances desired by the patient, or it failed, in which case there was little point in making further suicide attempts which had proved ineffective in the past. There were no other differentiating points of significance. It is questionable, therefore, whether one can distinguish between two populations of suicidal women by any means other than the fact that one group was pregnant and the other was not. On the evidence of this survey, it seems probable that the pregnancy was of relatively little importance and that the finding of 30 pregnant women in a large-scale survey of attempted suicide was a chance one.

It should not be forgotten, however, that the pregnant state was the main or contributory cause in 43% of the cases, so that pregnancy as such cannot be dismissed as wholly irrelevant. It will be recalled that in Otto's (1965) series of pregnant adolescents making suicide attempts, 43.6% gave pregnancy as the principal cause for their actions, although interpersonal conflict with lovers could scarcely be separated from the pregnancy as precipitants of attempted suicide. In Whitlock and Edward's (1968) series, 57% of the patients definitely wanted to have their babies, and it is interesting to note that the incidence of attempted suicide decreased after the second trimester. The fact that 53% of the pregnancies were conceived extramaritally or premaritally apparently made little difference to the patients' attitudes to the coming baby. The incidence of previous psychiatric care and previous suicide attempts seem to indicate that these patients did not differ significantly from the nonpregnant women and had features of personality and mental disorder which, more clearly than the pregnancy, were relevant to the suicidal acts. Over one third of the patients continued to show mental disturbances one year or more after their attempted suicides.

Few other investigations of suicidal behavior, unfortunately, have provided much information on the motivation of any pregnant patients included in these surveys. Harrington and Cross (1959) considered that suicidal behavior during pregnancy was not specifically related to the pregnancy. In their six cases, of 33 women aged 15–44, only one was single. On the other hand, four of five suicide attempts during pregnancy recorded by Sclare and Hamilton (1963) in Glasgow were considered to be related to the pregnancy, but no details of these five patients were given. Gabrielson et al (1970) studied 104 suicide attempts by adolescent girls. There were 14 examples of attempted suicide related to pregnancy, but only two of these apparently occurred during the pregnancy itself. The remainder were postpartum events.

Otto (1965), in his investigation of 1226 attempted suicide cases in adolescent females, found that 75 were pregnant, although not all knew it at the time. Thirty-three claimed the pregnancy to be the cause of the suicidal behavior, but most gave other reasons such as "love conflicts," family problems, and other difficulties. Mental illness was rarely a factor in this group of young women, and Otto considered that a steady relationship with the father at the time of the pregnancy was an important protection against suicidal behavior. Burke (1976), in her study of attempted suicide among West Indian immigrants in Birmingham, England, found that nine of 41 cases were pregnant. Burke considered that the pregnancy contributed to a situation already made stressful by unemployment, financial difficulties, and disputes with parents or lovers.

From these reports, a number of conclusions can be drawn. First, suicidal behavior during pregnancy is by no means invariably provoked solely by the pregnant state. It seems generally to be agreed that violent interpersonal disputes involving young, emotionally unstable women are more conducive to compulsive suicidal acts than the pregnancy itself. As far as can be ascertained, these impulsive acts occur more frequently in the early months of pregnancy, although this is by no means an invariable rule.

If all too little is known about suicidal attempts in pregnancy, and there is no reason to think that those coming to official notice constitute the total number, even less is known about those who succeed in taking their lives. Apart from those who commit suicide during the puerperium, often the consequence of a major psychotic illness, one might presume that some of those taking their lives during the last trimester are also suffering from severe mental disorders.

An unusual case was the patient who attempted suicide while actually in labor (Neale, 1976). She had a past history of epilepsy and was fearful lest a prophylactic injection against yellow fever during the pregnancy might have damaged the fetus. On recovery she showed no evidence of depression, and one can only speculate whether an ictal mood disturbance associated with hypertension had been sufficient to cause a transitory depression of such intensity as to make her feel that suicide was the only possible course available to her. An even more bizarre action was that taken by a 20-year-old married woman who, in the course of her second pregnancy, decided that at 17 weeks she did not wish to continue (Kloss, 1964). She "shot the baby" through her abdomen. The fetus was killed, but the mother survived. Remarkably few details of her mental state were given, but she was said to be depressed and responded well to tranylcypromine.

Particularly tragic are those young single women who, erroneously believing themselves to be pregnant, take their lives. One can only presume that in such cases the overwhelming effect of fear and anticipated shame is enough to cause such a drastic step to be taken.

This is not the place to discuss the pros and cons of termination of pregnancy on psychiatric grounds. However, each patient requires the fullest psychiatric assessment, and it would be foolish to dismiss suicidal threats as a reason for termination on the grounds that suicide in pregnancy does not occur. In fact, the evidence shows that, although it is rare, it undoubtedly does occur and as far as possible should be prevented.

SECTION III

TIMING, METHODS, AND HARM TO FETUS

CHAPTER 7

OVERVIEW OF TIMING, METHODS, AND HARM TO FETUS IN COMPLETED AND ATTEMPTED SUICIDE DURING PREGNANCY

GEORGE J. KLEINER
WILMA MARKUS GRESTON

It is difficult to obtain exact data, with specific details, on the timing and methods of completed and attempted suicide during pregnancy, primarily because of the lack of uniformity of reporting. This is in keeping with the difficulties encountered previously in collating the statistics on the incidence of suicide during pregnancy (Chapter 4). Despite the meager data, an attempt has been made to assemble it in a logical and sequential fashion.

TIMING

Completed Suicide

During pregnancy Most reports do not include detailed information as to precisely when the woman committed suicide during her pregnancy or the postpartum. Those reports which did indicate the timing of the suicide have been compiled (Figure 7-1). Some were reported in months, others in weeks. In an effort to present these figures with some uniformity, they have been converted to approximate weeks of pregnancy. The numbers are too small to warrant statistical significance, but perhaps point to a trend in relation to duration of pregnancy and suicide. In the two largest single groups of patients (Potondi, 1965; Weir, Chapter 5), suicide occurs more frequently in the first 12 weeks of pregnancy. From 13 to 28 weeks the differences between weeks are less marked, with the lowest levels being reached at 29–36 weeks. From these lowest levels, an increase in the incidence of suicide occurs in the last four weeks of pregnancy.

Another way to look at this might be to consider that 56 suicides took place in the first 20 weeks of pregnancy, whereas 40 occurred in the last 20 weeks.

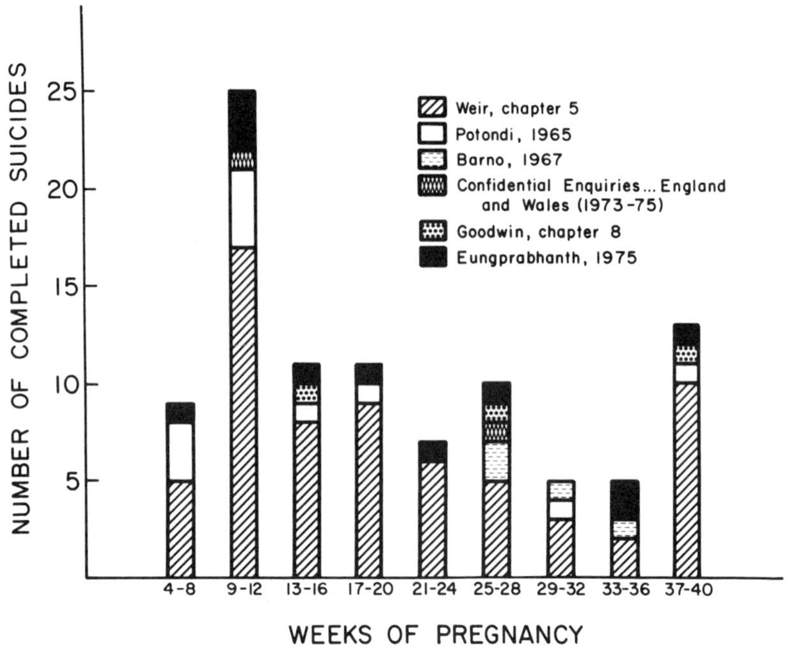

Figure 7-1 Timing of completed suicide in weeks of pregnancy.

Teleologically one could explain the tendency to commit suicide in terms of the psychologic moods of the pregnant woman during the specific trimesters of pregnancy (see Chapter 12 for additional discussion of this topic). In early pregnancy (up to 12 weeks), women occasionally decompensate, particularly those with anxiety problems, domestic difficulties, or psychiatric disease. This is reflected, for example, in the condition known as hyperemesis gravidarum or excessive vomiting of pregnancy (Deutsch, 1944–1945; Chertock, 1972). In this condition, the hormonal influences on the vomiting center of the brain as well as the psychological stresses of pregnancy are implicated. Interpersonal relationships or other domestic or environmental pressures contribute to the appearance of this syndrome. Similarly, it has been recognized that the middle part of pregnancy (13–28 weeks) is less stressful psychologically. There is a general feeling of well-being and confidence, even euphoria. It is interesting to speculate that the lessening of suicidal potential may be somewhat related to the growing maternal awareness of the fetus as a human being. Most women perceive fetal movement from the middle of pregnancy. It may be here that the ethic against murder comes into play, when the mother thinks about the fetus as a "real child" and recognizes its potential to survive. One could look at the last trimester of pregnancy (29–40 weeks) as a period when suicide is less likely to occur, with the exception of the well-recognized period of preterm anxiety that women exhibit just prior to the end of pregnancy. The relative increase in the number of suicides at 37–40 weeks, as seen on the bar graph (Figure 7-1) could be interpreted as reflecting this stress.

Labor Completed suicide in the course of labor is almost unknown. Woodis and Robinson (1960), in reviewing literature relative to their case report of attempted suicide during the course of labor, quote Von Sury from an article published in 1908. Von Sury reported on two cases of completed suicide during labor; according to Woodis and Robinson, these appear to be the only two cases of completed suicide during labor in the world literature. One additional case is reported elsewhere in this book by Weir (Chapter 5), who describes a woman (Mrs. B.K.) who was in labor when she committed suicide. There have been reports of attempted suicide in labor, but these, also, are exceedingly rare (Von Sury, 1908; Woodis and Robinson, 1960; Neale, 1976).

Postpartum Only meager information regarding the precise time of suicide during the postpartum period is available. Although mention of postpartum suicide may be made in other articles, only three gave sufficiently detailed data to be put into tabular form. All women reported by Barno (1967) over a 15-year period in Minnesota, who committed suicide in the postpartum, did so in the first three months (Table 7-1). Evaluation by a psychiatric consultant of the case protocols indicates that two suffered from schizophrenia and eight from psychiatric depression, but most neither sought nor received psychiatric care. Goodwin (Chapter 8) describes three cases of suicide in the first postpartum year, one of which was within the first three months after delivery.

Reports on Confidential Enquiries into Maternal Deaths in England and Wales (1952–1954; 1955–1957; 1958–1960; 1961–1963; 1964–1966; 1967–1969; 1970–1972; 1973–1975) mentioned postpartum suicides in the years 1969–1975 inclusive. Between 1967 and 1969, among 13 women who died in the postpartum period, eight gave a history of mental disorder or at least one previous suicide attempt. There was no identification as to when the suicide occurred. Of 11 deaths reported in 1970–1972, one was postabortal and 10 followed delivery, but, again, no specific time during the postpartum was mentioned. Seven of the women committed suicide more than six weeks after the delivery. In five cases there was evidence of puerperal depression. One of the women was charged with infanticide. Of the 12 women who died postpartum during 1973–1975, 10 deaths occurred more than six weeks after the delivery (Table 7-1). Five of the nine patients who killed themselves between six weeks and 11 months postpartum had long psychiatric histories. One other had been treated for depression prior to the suicide. Another patient was admitted to the psychiatric unit three weeks after delivery with depression from which she apparently recovered, only to commit suicide

Table 7-1
Postpartum Suicides

Source	Months Postpartum 3	3–4	7–12
Barno (1967)	10	0	0
England and Wales*	2	2	8
Goodwin†	1	0	2

*Reports on Confidential Enquiries into Maternal Deaths in England and Wales (1973–1975).
†See Chapter 8.

four months after the delivery. The other two patients apparently had not given any signs of psychiatric illness. These figures from the Confidential Enquiries into Maternal Deaths in England and Wales are especially noteworthy, as they appear in such contrast to Sim's (1963) study which was derived from a psychiatric hospital in a large English city.

It is of particular interest that, of the 14 women who committed suicide (two during pregnancy and 12 after delivery), four were of Asian origin. Three died 16 days, 3 months, and 6½ months after delivery. This is a relatively high proportion when compared to the indigenous population of England and Wales. In a similar vein, Dr. A.L. Becker, previously principal psychiatrist in the Department of Psychiatry at the University of the Witwatersrand Medical School and Johannesburg Hospital (written communication, May 1983) acknowledged the rarity of suicide by white-skinned women in South Africa in association with unwanted pregnancy. However, he pointed out that in Durban, South Africa, where there is a large Indian population, illegitimate pregnancy in unmarried girls is the main cause for attempted or completed suicide among women of childbearing age. How curious that, both in England (and Wales) and South Africa, a group of Asian women appears to be singled out in the statistics of suicide during pregnancy. One could propose that perhaps some environmental stresses, such as social alienation and language isolation, influence immigrants. Another factor could be the cultural and religious predisposition of Asian women to commit suicide (Kleiner and Greston, Chapter 3). However, no reports appear in the Western literature which would indicate a similar phenomenon on the Indian subcontinent. Barbara Snyder (1977), in her article on the importance of cultural factors in suicide studies, pointed out the need for an awareness of and sensitivity to cultural factors that affect the suicide rate. She suggested that examination of cultural factors that contribute to individual stress and of cultural phenomena undergoing rapid change might be an aid to those involved in suicide studies.

Postpartum psychosis In the past, it generally has been accepted that postpartum psychosis greatly increases the risk of suicide. A lesser form of depression, the so-called "blue period" which occurs in the early puerperium, is common (see Chapters 12, 14, and 15). The severe form of postpartum depression which expresses itself in the form of psychosis could lead to suicide or assault on the child or both. A critical overview of the literature leads one to believe that it is rare and even less likely to occur than generally was given credence in the past.

In Sim's (1963) study from Birmingham, of the 213 patients who had postpartum psychosis severe enough to be committed to psychiatric hospitals, none completed or even attempted suicide. No report on suicide in the postpartum period was found in the New York City Department of Health (1983) data, despite the fact that maternal death is so defined by law in New York City as to include both duration of pregnancy and the subsequent 90 days of the postpartum period; this may be a reflection of the difficulties of data collection.

Although uncommon, there are occasional reports of completed suicide in the postpartum period, especially if the entire first year after delivery is included. For example, Astrachan (Chapter 15) notes three instances of attempted suicide in 13 patients with severe psychologic disorders of the puerperium who were studied in depth in a New York City hospital. Similarly, Destounis (Chapter 13), in his discussion on postpartum psychiatric syndromes, describes a woman with a severe psychotic reaction leading to a serious attempt at suicide. As mentioned elsewhere (Chapter 4), there was a newspaper report (Fay and Meskil, 1983) of a mother in New York City who, after drowning her 12-day-old baby, placed it in a drawer. Her father tried unsuccessfully to revive his grandchild. Before the psychiatrist who had been treating the 31-year-old woman arrived, she plunged to her death from a fifth-story window. She had been married and divorced, her ex-husband apparently was not the baby's father, and she had a history of psychiatric problems.

Anniversary reaction Another variant of postpartum psychosis could be the so-called "anniversary reaction." Although no completed suicides were reported, Tishler (1981) described two adolescents who, following elective abortion, attempted suicide on the approximate date on which the baby would have been born. Both girls had involved psychiatric histories which might have increased their vulnerability to emotional stress and potential suicide.

Attempted Suicide

Only sporadic articles on attempted suicide may be found. These case reports, when present, were derived from the need to describe an unusual damage in combination with the suicide attempt, but attempted suicide was not the primary motivation for publication. For example, Battle and Marshall (1952) described a case in which the patient's history was typical of an acute puerperal depression after the birth of her second child. Following an earlier suicide attempt by gas poisoning, the 30-year-old woman set her nightgown on fire during a second unsuccessful attempt at gassing herself. The body of the report, however, described the severe burns which were sustained and the medical and psychiatric management.

There is surprisingly little detailed information about attempted suicide. The only careful observations were those described by Otto (1965) and Whitlock (Chapter 6). Otto (1965) investigated suicide attempts in Sweden made by pregnant women under 21 years of age. Duration of pregnancy was recorded in calendar months. Almost half of these 43 women made suicide attempts during the first three calendar months of pregnancy (Figure 7-2). From the third to the ninth calendar months, on the average, there was a sustained decrease in the incidence of attempted suicide, except for a rise in the seventh month. This very much resembles the timing previously noted for completed suicide, except, in the latter, there appeared a significant rise at the very end of pregnancy (Figure 7-1). The number of patients in Figures 7-1 and 7-2 is so small,

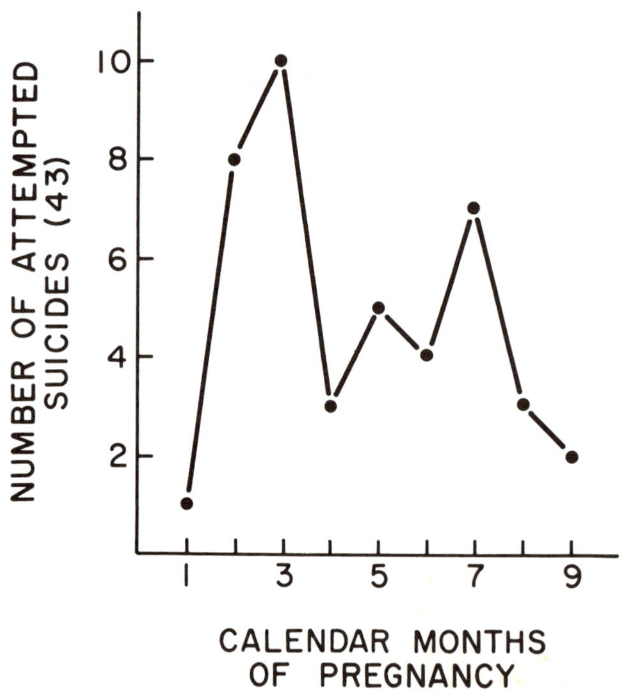

Figure 7-2 Timing of attempted suicide in calendar months of pregnancy (modified from Otto, 1965).

however, that one should be cautious about overinterpreting the differences, but there does appear to be a similar trend.

In order to compare Otto's (1965) with Whitlock's (Chapter 6) data on attempted suicide, Otto's calendar months of pregnancy were converted to first (up to 12 weeks), second (13–28 weeks), and third (29–40 weeks) trimesters. As can be seen in Figure 7-3, the ratio of suicides during each trimester was very similar, ie, the majority of suicides occurring in the first and second trimesters with only a few attempts made in the last trimester of pregnancy.

Menstrual Cycle

There is some evidence that women, falsely believing themselves pregnant, commit suicide when their amenorrhea or lack of menstruation actually is due to other disturbances and not to pregnancy (Sim, 1963; Goodwin, Chapters 2 and 8). It is possible to postulate that those women who have irregular periods, with a longer cycle, could think themselves pregnant, when in fact the attempted or completed suicide could be provoked by the physiologic and psychologic stresses of the premenstruum (Dalton, 1959, 1961; MacKinnon et al, 1959). It is possible that this phenomenon could be explained on the basis of hormonal

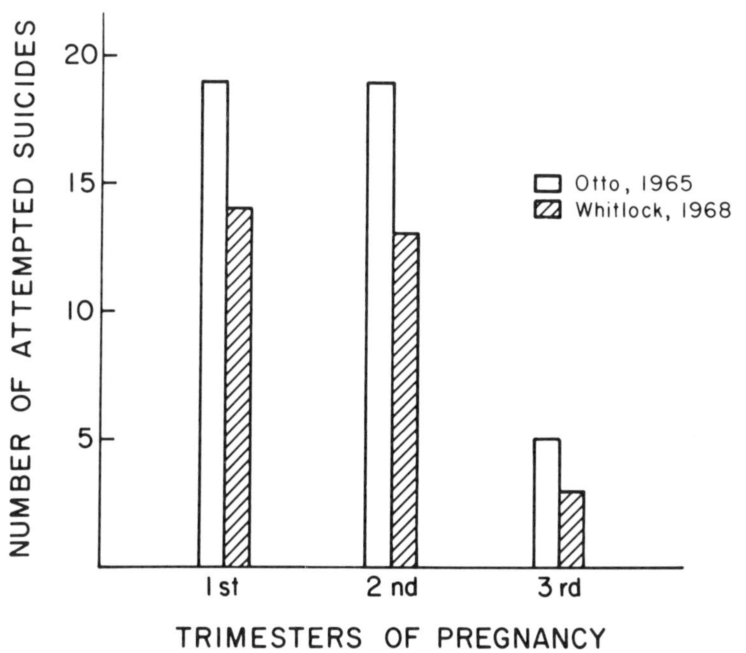

Figure 7-3 Timing of attempted suicide in trimesters of pregnancy.

changes, in particular, the reduction of circulating estrogen. In lesser measure, this is similar to the sudden reduction of that hormone in the postpartum, which is associated with depression (Saks, Chapter 13).

MacKinnon et al (1959), however, in their article on the lethal hazards of the luteal phase of the menstrual cycle showed that most of the suicides which occurred in women between the ages of 18 and 46 did so in mid-luteal rather than late luteal phase, when the level of estrogen was still relatively high and the progesterone was at its peak.

One has to seriously consider Dalton's (1959) evidence that a relationship exists between acute psychiatric hospital admissions and the menstrual cycle. Her investigation into the time of admission of 276 psychiatric patients emphasized the importance of menstruation and the premenstruum in relation to the onset of acute psychiatric episodes. She stated that "46% of all admissions occurred during this time. Indeed, 53% of attempted suicides, 47% of patients with depression, and 47% of schizophrenic patients were admitted during menstruation or the premenstruum." Mandell and Mandell (1967) collected data from the Los Angeles Suicide Prevention Center. They confirmed Dalton's (1959) findings "regarding times of maximum psychological disturbance during the menstrual cycle: during early menstruation, premenstrually, and midcycle (in that order)."

Dalton (1961) also felt that there were specific hormonal changes which caused women to commit crime during menstruation and the premenstruum. She stated that "premenstrual tension is also accompanied by irritability, lethargy, depression, and water retention, and these symptoms alone may be responsible for certain crimes—for example, irritability and loss of temper may lead to violence and assault, lethargy may lead to child neglect, and depression to suicide."

A similar correlation was implied by Ribeiro (1962), in a letter to the editor of the *British Medical Journal*. He related an interesting observation on postmortem examinations of 26 women in Kenya who committed suicide. Twenty-two were Hindu women who committed suicide by pouring kerosene over themselves and setting themselves on fire, one European took sleeping pills, and three Africans hung themselves. Twenty-three of the 26 women were menstruating at the time of their death and two were pregnant.

Although many others (Dalton, 1959; MacKinnon et al, 1959; Ribeiro, 1962; Mandell and Mandell, 1967) found that suicide or attempted suicide correlated with the menstrual cycle, there is "no general agreement as to the time of the cycle when women are most liable to emotional upset" (Birtchnell and Floyd, 1974). In an effort to establish whether women attempted suicide more at certain times during the menstrual cycle than at others, Birtchnell and Floyd (1974) studied all cases of attempted suicide received in the accident and emergency department of a district general hospital in Chichester, England. It is sobering that they reached a negative conclusion in this critical study of attempted suicide and the menstrual cycle. Of particular interest is their additional comment that, of 76 women, 13 were either pregnant or beyond the expected date of the next menstrual period when they attempted suicide. These were predominantly young, unmarried women. Birtchnell and Floyd (1974) felt that the suicidal behavior might be associated with a woman knowing or fearing she was pregnant and that emotional disturbances can influence the duration of the menstrual cycle. In fact, it has been recognized that many of the antipsychotic drugs may be associated with secondary amenorrhea in some women, and thus could be responsible for lengthening of the menstrual cycle, possibly leading to a misinterpretation of early pregnancy.

METHODS

There is little consistent information on the means by which women kill themselves during pregnancy, except for isolated detailed studies. Although the numbers in individual reports may be small, they have been tabulated in an attempt to summarize the available information (Table 7-2). The most common methods of committing suicide, both during pregnancy and the postpartum, were the ingestion of an overdose of barbiturates and allied drugs and by gas poisoning. Violent deaths (intentional auto crash, jumping from heights or in front of moving vehicles, cutting of wrists or throat), drowning, use of firearms, and hanging were also employed. Certain geographic areas favor one method over another. For instance, at that time, gas was the most prevalent choice in England (1943–1962) and in Hungary (1965), while guns seem to be preferred in the state of New Mexico in the United States (1983). It is surprising to note that hanging was relatively uncommon. It appears from Weir's (Chapter 5) detailed analysis that there is not a significant difference in women in the choice of method of committing suicide whether or not one is pregnant (Chapter 5, Figure 5-1). The availability of the killing instrument or the opportunity appears to be of paramount importance in determining the method used.

Methodology may also be related to the cultural or ethnic background of the woman who commits suicide. For instance, Gelfand (1976) pointed out that the most usual method of suicide in the Black African in Rhodesia was by hanging. However, in those of European descent living in the same area, the most usual method of suicide was by shooting, poisoning, and taking drugs. Ribeiro (1962) observed that pouring kerosene and setting themselves on fire was the favorite method among the Hindu women in Kenya.

Further discussion of methods of suicide during pregnancy and the postpartum can be found in the articles by Goodwin, Weir, Whitlock, and Rosenberg in Chapters 2 and 8, 5, 6, and 9, respectively.

Table 7-2
Methods of Suicide in Women during Pregnancy and Postpartum

Source	Total Suicides	Overdose		Gas	Drowning	Hanging	Guns	Violent*	Unknown
		Barbiturates	*Other Drugs and Toxins*						
Completed									
Bengtsson, 1947 Sweden	19	—	15	—	1	1	1	—	1
Potondi, 1965 Hungary	11	2	2	6	—	—	—	1	—
OSMA Committee, 1966 Ohio, USA	3	—	—	1	1	—	1	—	—
Barno, 1967 Minnesota, USA	14	2	—	1	3	1	3	4	—
Eungprabhanth, 1975 Thailand	11	—	7	—	1	3	—	—	—
OSMA Committee, 1976 Ohio, USA	3	—	—	—	1	—	1	1	—
Dept. of Health, 1983 New York City, USA	7	—	2	—	—	—	—	3	2
Weir, Chapter 5 London, England	65	13	4	32	7	1	—	7	1
Goodwin, Chapter 8 New Mexico, USA	8	1	—	1	—	1	5	—	—
Rosenberg, Chapter 9 California, USA	3	—	—	—	—	—	1	2	—
Total	144	18	30	41	14	7	12	18	4
Attempted									
Woodis and Robinson, 1960 England	9	1	—	5	—	1	—	2	—
Whitlock and Edwards, 1968 Australia	30	23	6	—	—	—	—	1	—
Total	39	24	6	5	—	1	—	3	—
Combined Total	183	42	36	46	14	8	12	21	4

*Auto crash, jumping from heights and/or in front of moving vehicles, cutting one's wrist or throat.

HARM TO THE FETUS

Another consideration for discussion on suicide and attempted suicide in pregnant women is the possible effect on the baby. It is important to consider the disturbance of maternal health and the possible noxious effects on the developing or growing fetus in those women who survived the suicide attempt and in whom the pregnancy continued to viable delivery. One could readily postulate that a serious attempt on her life by a pregnant woman could result in some fetal damage. It is necessary, therefore, to carefully annotate the type of harmful substances, the duration of exposure, and their effect on the mother.

If an attempted suicide occurs very early in pregnancy, there may be an effect on somatogenesis, as well as suspected behavioral teratogenesis (Golub and Golub, 1981). For example, a significant number of women who attempt to commit suicide are psychiatrically disturbed and, not infrequently, are placed on psychotropic drugs. The use of antipsychotic drugs during pregnancy has been reviewed by Tylden (1977), Lewis (1978), Golub and Golub (1981), and Sriwatanakal and Weis (1982); attempted suicide with these readily available medications could take place. Most psychotropic drugs or tranquilizers have been detected in the fetal circulation of experimental animals and have caused teratogenic effects (Szabo and Brent, 1974). Between the second and seventh week of gestation is the period of organogenesis, and that is the time when the developing embryo is most sensitive to teratogenic effects of the drugs. This sensitive period may be even longer, as it is known that natural diseases such as rubella (German measles) have affected fetuses even as late as 16 weeks of gestation, causing significant congenital abnormalities (Miller et al, 1982). There is still some controversy dealing specifically with antipsychotic drugs, as there are several other control studies which have shown no increase in the ratio of congenital abnormalities in the infants of mothers who have taken these medications during the first 12 weeks of intrauterine life (Sobel, 1960; Shader and DiMascio, 1970).

When attempted suicide occurs later in the pregnancy, it could possibly affect the intrauterine environment and damage the growing fetus directly. The type of damage basically depends on the type of insult (chemical or physical). For example, ingestion of large doses of drugs (which cross the placental barrier) affect the fetus in a manner similar to the mother. The concept of a "placental barrier" is no longer supported by most investigators; in fact, it is looked upon as a "placental sieve" (Sriwatanakal and Weis, 1982). The current belief is that drugs cross the placenta primarily by passive diffusion (Asiling and Way, 1971). It has been shown by Goldberg and DiMascio (1976) and Wadell and Marlow (1981) that lipid soluble drugs which did not ionize easily passed readily to the fetus and from it back to the mother. Those drugs that were highly ionized or had low lipid solubility, if they did cross the placenta, did so with some difficulty. But the principle should be kept in mind that any medication, chemical, or toxin given to or taken by the pregnant women may be transferred across the placental barrier to the fetus to a varying degree.

In addition to damaging the growing fetus directly, a suicide attempt later in pregnancy may affect the fetal physiologic function. For instance, in a case report of acute maternal arsenic intoxication, Lugo and associates (1969) described a 17-year-old married white mother (gravida 3, para 1, abortus 1) who ingested rat poison containing inorganic arsenic. Although she survived the suicide attempt, the child died at 11 hours of age. Prematurity (seven months) and hyaline membrane disease might have been the major causes of death, but Lugo et al (1969) suspected that the severe intraalveolar hemorrhage and extremely high arsenic levels found at autopsy in liver, brain, and kidneys played a role.

It has also been recognized that young females, many of whom were unmarried women who mentioned pregnancy or fear of pregnancy as the reason, attempted suicide by ingestion of analgesic or soporific drugs as the preferred method (Nashold, 1965). Jacobziner (1965), describing suicide during adolescence (ages 12–20) in New York City, indicated that illegitimate pregnancy was the reason for the suicide attempt with chemical agents in 4.8%. In these girls, the most common toxic products were aspirins (35%), barbiturates (33%), tranquilizers (12%), and nonbarbiturate drugs (9.5%). He pointed out that the use of these agents was "undoubtedly related to the degree of availability and accessibility in the home."

If a woman attempts suicide with gas poisoning or any manner where her oxygenation is reduced, it would result in similar shortcomings in the fetus. This could lead either to intrauterine death or some degree of permanent brain damage due to prolonged intrauterine hypoxia.

Physical trauma to the mother may result in direct damage to the uterus, placenta, and/or fetus. For example, gunshot wounds, cutting wrist or throat, jumping from heights, intentional automobile accidents, and other forms of violent self-destruction could result in blood loss, separation of the placenta, and maternal shock, again leading to a compromised intrauterine environment directly or indirectly. The extent and duration of hemorrhage, loss of consciousness, or any maternal trauma should be noted and resuscitative measures described in detail in case of any possible future effect on the baby.

Perhaps the most significant and dangerous effect of attempted suicide is that it could lead to premature labor, as most suicide attempts take place before term. If the baby is born alive, it most likely would be immature or premature, an especially lethal factor which markedly reduces its chances for survival (Pritchard and MacDonald, 1980). In addition, the baby may be secondarily affected by the trauma, toxic effects of ingested poisons or drugs, or by the resuscitative efforts to save the mother.

A variety of possible combinations of outcomes of suicide attempts have been reported. In one of the rare instances of a report of attempted suicide in labor (Neale, 1976), both mother and baby survived after an overdose of diazepam and amylobarbitone. The mother was initially unconscious but recovered sufficiently to deliver a live baby; thereafter she made good progress. Although the baby cried at birth and required only routine resuscitation, his breathing was shallow and irregular, he remained cold, hypotonic, and areflexic. It took 48 hours for the infant to recover the sucking reflex and begin gradual bottle feeding. In some cases, the mother survived but the baby died, as was the case of arsenic poisoning (Lugo et al, 1969). Sometimes, the reverse was true: the mother died but the baby survived. Richard and Brooks (1966) described a case of poisoning with ferrous sulfate at 30 weeks of pregnancy. Although the mother died from hepatocellular damage from the iron poisoning, the baby survived despite a poor start at birth and prematurity. It is interesting to note the method of attempted suicide in this particular case, as ferrous sulfate is not usually suspected by the physician as a potential toxin. In fact, it is routinely given as an iron supplement for prevention of anemia to most pregnant women and is also available in similar dosages in some prenatal multivitamins which are obtainable without a prescription.

In terms of delayed effect, it has been suggested that children of mothers who attempted suicide should be followed for child neglect and even abuse (Gabrielson, Chapter 11; Suicide Risk in Teenage Pregnancy, 1971). This may be particularly true for women with previous psychiatric problems. Brown and Palmer (1975) described nine schizophrenic women who murdered their children. These women had been preoccupied with suicide before and after the murder. They pointed out that "all the women openly neglected their health and failed to seek proper medical attention during their pregnancy. Four had attempted selfabortions of the child they later murdered; seven had difficulty during labor during that birth, and seven suffered from postpartum depression. Five of those women had not shown postpartum symptoms after births of their other children. All of the women neglected their children, and several children were injured as a result."

In reviewing the potential physical and psychologic effects on the fetus or the baby in those women who attempted suicide while pregnant, it appears mandatory to carefully annotate details of the history and management of such patients. Once born, the child should be observed for the more obvious congenital abnormalities and after-effects resulting from the method of the attempt, and, also, for less discernible effects.

These might include such things as intellectual and emotional deprivation, numerous "accidents," as well as overt child abuse. In order to discover these handicaps early or to prevent harm to the child, it would be ideal to provide such a woman and her child with in-depth social service support and medical care for a prolonged period of time.

CHAPTER 8

THE MEANING AND THE MADNESS IN THE METHOD OF SUICIDE IN PREGNANCY: Contemporary Cases

JEAN GOODWIN

METHODS USED IN CONTEMPORARY SUICIDES IN PREGNANCY AS CLUES TO THE DEVELOPMENTAL MEANING OF THE ACT

In order to identify cases of suicide in pregnancy, I reviewed the 47 cases of suicide in women aged 15 to 44 which were reported to the New Mexico Medical Investigator in 1975 and in 1976. Of these 47 cases, only 14 had been autopsied, and in two of these autopsies, no information about reproductive organs was noted. The neglect at autopsy of the reproductive organs in cases of traumatic death has been noted previously (Maternal Mortality Committee, 1953). So, letters were sent to the physician and/or hospital listed on the death certificate, asking for medical records which would indicate the woman's pregnancy status at the time of death. In this way, reliable information about pregnancy status was obtained for 23 of the 47 suicides. In addition, I searched computerized records of New Mexico births, and stillbirths for 1974, 1975, and 1976 to determine if any of the women in the sample had given birth in those years. The stillbirth records revealed one maternal suicide which simply had not been reported to the medical investigator.

One thing that became clear in the search for information about this handful of suicides was that a pattern of concealment, both of the suicidal nature of the death, and of the woman's pregnancy, was as effective in real life as it was in the fictitious suicide of Maeve O'Riorden (Chapter 2). As noted above, one suicide was found which was registered as suicide on the death certificate but not reported to the medical investigator. Another death which occurred during the study period was ruled an accident with the following explanation: "She would not have done it on purpose because she thought she was pregnant." This pseudopregnant woman, six months postpartum, had been found in her garage, dead of carbon monoxide poisoning. This death was subsequently judged a suicide. When such a death is recognized as suicide, postpartum or pregnancy status is often not determined. Of the 47 women in the original sample, two were pseudopregnant, two were pregnant, and two were within the first year postpartum. In addition to these six, I investigated the suicide in pregnancy which had not been reported, and the postpartum, pseudopregnant suicide, which had originally been ruled accidental death. In only two of these eight cases were both the suicide and the pregnancy status accurately reported on the death certificate. In one of the two accurately reported cases the woman, who was eight months pregnant and who had attempted suicide earlier in the pregnancy, barricaded herself in her room, overdosed, and died, leaving a suicide note (see Contemporary Case Examples . . . , Late Pregnancy, later in this chapter). In the other accurately reported case, a woman who was 10 months postpartum and who had consulted a psychiatrist previously, shot her infant through the head and then herself. It would seem that a pregnant or postpartum suicide must make a deliberate statement in her death, both that she is suiciding and that pregnancy status is a factor, if her death certificate is to register this fact.

It is unclear how much of the "protective" effect of pregnancy against suicide is due to the protective efforts of families, friends, and physicians against recognizing and reporting suicides in pregnancy. Other epidemiological factors may contribute to a spurious "protective" effect. For example, within the age group 15–44, women aged 35–44 are at the highest risk for suicide and at the lowest risk for pregnancy. (In New Mexico only 6% of pregnancies occur in women over 35.) Most studies of suicides in pregnancy have looked at women in the age range 15–50 (Maternal Mortality Committee, 1953; Sim, 1963; Rosenberg and Silver, 1965; Resnik, 1971), and this even more distortingly inflates the denominator (total female suicides) with women unlikely to be pregnant; this yields a falsely low percentage of pregnancies among female suicides. The age group 15–34 is probably the most appropriate to study if one wants an accurate estimate of the percentage of pregnant women among female suicides. Using our coroner's data, and omitting the unreported suicide in pregnancy, and using as the denominator reported female suicides ages 15–34, we would have found that over 6% (2/32) were pregnant. Had we used ages 15–50, we would have found that only 3% (2/59) were pregnant. Another artifactual source for the "protective" effect of pregnancy is that single, divorced, and childless people are at higher risk for suicide (Veevers, 1973). It may be the social skills that lead to impregnation, rather than the pregnancy itself, which are protective against suicide.

Table 8-1 lists some of the characteristics of the eight pregnancy-related suicides found in this New Mexico study. Three of the eight women falsely believed themselves to be pregnant. This finding is contrary to the

Table 8-1
Characteristics of Pregnancy-Associated Suicides in New Mexico

Case	Pregnancy Status	Age	Marital Status	Method
1	Falsely believed herself pregnant; lutein cyst; consulted psychiatrist	20	M	Gunshot, head
2	Falsely believed herself pregnant; pituitary micro-adenoma; consulted psychiatrist	26	M	Hanging
3	14 weeks pregnant (not reported as suicide)	22	M	Gunshot, head
4	26 weeks pregnant	20	M	Gunshot, head
5	37 weeks pregnant; prior attempt 2nd trimester (refused psychiatric consultation)	24	M	Sedative overdose
6	6 weeks postpartum	25	M	Gunshot, head
7	7 months pregnant; also pseudopregnant 2nd trimester (not reported as suicide); consulted psychiatrist	28	M	Carbon monoxide, ? accident
8	10 months postpartum; complex suicide: also killed infant; consulted psychiatrist	30	M	Gunshot, head

Western cultural belief, fostered by the medical community, that pregnancy is a clearly definable, all-or-none entity (Silverblatt and Goodwin, 1981). However, one study of the menstrual cycles of women who attempt suicide (Birtchnell and Floyd, 1975) indicates that uncertainty about pregnancy is not unusual in this group. This study found that 13 (11.8%) of the attempters made the suicide attempt at a time when their next menstrual period was overdue. Nine of these 13 (or 8.4% of all suicide attempters) believed they were pregnant at the time of the attempt; four actually were pregnant. When 110 age-matched controls from a general population sample were interviewed, it was found that only three (2.7%) of these women were beyond the date when their next period was due. None of the controls believed themselves to be pregnant.

The three pseudopregnant women in the New Mexico sample (cases 1, 2, and 7 in Table 8-1) had been confused in various ways about their pregnancy status. The postpartum woman had been confirmed as pregnant by her physician after what was, in retrospect, a false-positive pregnancy test. A second woman had been discharged from a psychiatric hospital and had shot herself before the negative results of a pregnancy test returned from the laboratory; autopsy revealed a lutein cyst of the ovary (see Contemporary Case Examples . . . , Pseudopregnancy, later in this chapter). The third pseudopregnant woman had been treated for pituitary microadenoma, but had left treatment and had told her family that she was pregnant before hanging herself. All three women had previously consulted psychiatrists, and all had been diagnosed as having personality disorders. It is likely that their psychiatric diagnoses interfered with their ability to perceive accurately pregnancy status, as well as interfering with their ability to cope with a possible pregnancy. All three women were involved in stormy marriages with repeated separations. The false pregnancy may have been an unconscious attempt to stabilize the marital relationship, but one which increased the woman's suicidal despair when marital upsets continued.

Two of the three women who were actually pregnant at the time of the suicide shot themselves in the head in their homes after an argument with the husband, at a time when the pregnancy was becoming obvious. The third woman had made a suicide attempt by overdose in the second trimester, but completed suicide by sedative overdose when she was eight months pregnant. Two of the three postpartum suicides also resulted from gunshot wounds to the head. Only one of the eight women in Table 8-1 died by overdose, and her barricading of her door added a touch of violence to that method.

All eight were married. As in the literary cases (Chapter 2), it may be that the acceptability of paternal support, not merely its availability, is the important factor. Teenage suicides are notably absent. As in the literary suicides, these suicidal women were old enough to have accumulated losses, failures, and disappointments.

Is the New Mexico experience unique? Two previous studies (Rosenberg and Silver, 1965; Barno, 1967) done in the United States described seven cases of suicide in pregnancy. This study added three cases. Of the total of 10 women who committed suicide in pregnancy, nine were married, nine were in the second or third trimester of pregnancy, and seven used a relatively violent method—jumping, carbon monoxide, or gunshot. Only one was a teen-ager. Of the six suicides for which motive and place of death were recorded, all took place in the home after an argument with the husband.

This pattern contrasts with the findings in women who unsuccessfully attempt suicide in pregnancy (Whitlock and Edwards, 1968). Table 8-2 shows that unsuccessful attempts tend to occur in unmarried women in the first trimester. Almost all such attempts are by overdose. Many are interpreted as manipulative efforts to alter the environment to accommodate a problem pregnancy.

Table 8-2
Characteristics of Suicidal Behavior in First, Second, and Third Trimesters of Pregnancy

	Married	Trimester	Method	Place	Motive
30 unsuccessful suicide attempts in pregnancy*	No (16/30;53%)	1 (14/30;47%)	Overdose (29/30;97%)	? (23/30;77%)	After argument
Maeve O'Riorden	No	1	Overdose	Home	Conceal pregnancy
Hedda Gabler	Yes	1–2	Gunshot	Home	Rejection by husband
10 completed suicides in pregnancy from the USA*	Yes (9/10;90%)	2–3 (9/10;90%)	Violent (7/10;70%)	Home (6/6 where data available)	Rejection by husband (6/6 where data available)
Jeanne Hebuterne	Yes (common law)	3	Jump	Home	Death of husband

*See Whitlock and Edwards (1968) for data about attempts, and Goodwin and Harris (1979), Rosenberg and Silver (1965), and Barno (1967) for data about completed suicides.

Using Table 8-2, one can begin to integrate patterns of suicidal behavior at various stages of pregnancy with the developmental tasks of pregnancy. Early in pregnancy, the pregnant woman attempts to cope with the reality of the pregnancy and to make the basic adjustments that will be necessary (Jessner et al, 1970). Potentially reversible methods, as chosen by Maeve O'Riorden and by the majority of "unsuccessful" attempters, are consistent with this developmental need to elicit an environmental response to an internal crisis.

As the pregnancy becomes obvious, a crisis of identity is added to the crisis of adaptation. Like Hedda Gabler, the pregnant woman becomes aware that pregnancy threatens masculine and regressive elements of her identity. Hedda Gabler's insistence on playing with her father's dueling pistols, even in dangerous and self-destructive ways, is most sympathetic as an assertion of her right to retain these masculine aspects of her identity. One wonders if her revulsion at suicide by gunshot to the abdomen is defensive against unconscious fantasies about killing the troublesome fetus with her dueling pistol in a direct infanticide. Gunshot to the abdomen has in fact been reported as a method of criminal abortion (Takki et al, 1969; Thonet, 1967; Kloss, 1964).

In the last trimester of pregnancy (Goodwin and Jaramillo, 1981), the burdensome weight of the fetus and the associated bodily changes in the mother lead her intrapsychic life into fantasies about the self as monster or the fetus as monster. Dread of delivery, with its threat of pain, violence, and death, colors these developmental preoccupations. Overdose may again be chosen as the suicide method in the last trimester, because sedation is sought to calm frightening fantasies and to delay the inevitable moment of delivery. At this point in pregnancy, it is obvious that the mother's suicide involves a homicide as well. Like Jeanne Hebuterne, the woman who kills herself in late pregnancy may seek out a method that is aesthetically satisfying and that substitutes an angelic transformation for the monstrous transformation that she fears. She may also seek a method, like Hebuterne's angelic fall, that emphasizes her fantasy that death is the only way of rescuing and of restoring herself and her child to a better world in which separation is not a threat.

The next phase in this continuum of pregnancy-related suicidal behavior involves suicidal and infanticidal behaviors in the postpartum period. Barno (1967), who found only four suicides in pregnancy in his study of over 300,000 live births, found 10 suicides in the first three months postpartum. All were by violent means—gunshot wound, hanging, cutting of the throat, drowning, auto crash, and jumping in front of a train. This is in rough agreement with data about postpartum psychoses which indicate that only one fifth of such psychosis begin during the pregnancy and that the increased risk for psychosis continues to the end of the first postpartum year (Thomas and Gordon, 1959; Pugh et al,

1963). Although delivery allows maternal suicide and infanticide to be separated once again, fantasies of infanticide are almost universal in postpartum suicides and vice versa. In about 60% of cases, the woman who kills her infant has also planned her own suicide (Rodenbury, 1971). Later child abuse is similarly associated with suicidal behavior in the parent (Goodwin, 1981).

The psychological connection between infanticide and suicide may account for some of the suicidal ideation that occurs when women seek legal abortion (Otto, 1966; Fischer, 1974). Even though infanticide without suicide is technically possible in the first half of pregnancy and in the postpartum period, for some women it may not be psychologically possible to contemplate the one without the other.

Postpartum infanticides and suicides have been linked in several traditions to hostility toward the child's father and to a desire for revenge against him. In Greek mythology, Medea, when her husband Jason abandons her for another woman, avenges herself by killing their two sons (Stern, 1978). Medea had earlier betrayed her own father to help Jason to acquire the Golden Fleece. La Malinche is another woman who betrays her own Indian people to become the translator and mistress of the invading Cortes. Folk legends say that she killed herself and her children when Cortes left Mexico to marry a Spanish lady and that she still roams the region as a malevolent ghost, tempting others to suicide and killing other children (Hawes, 1968). Madame Butterfly (Feggetter, 1980), whose family had deserted her when she married Pinkerton, is able to relinquish her child to Pinkerton when he, too, abandons her, and kills only herself. However, a double suicide of mother and child, or shinju (Kleiner, 1979), might have been the solution chosen by a less altruistic Japanese teenager in similar circumstances. All of these postpartum fables describe elements seen in intrapartum suicidal/infanticidal behavior: isolation from the original family, abandonment by the husband, and anger with the husband that is expressed in a tragic but dramatic act of violence. Since most patriarchal societies treat children as the property of the father, the mother's destruction of the father's child directly questions and defies this power and spitefully hurts and deprives the husband.

CONTEMPORARY CASE EXAMPLES ILLUSTRATING THE SPECTRUM OF METHODS IN PREGNANCY-RELATED SUICIDES: A REPRISE

Table 8-2 combines statistical data with literary and biographical cases to describe the spectrum of suicidal behaviors as they relate to developmental risks at each stage of pregnancy.

The following contemporary case histories allow the reader to review and reintegrate the conflicts and motivations that are revealed by the suicide method. These cases review the previously discussed themes of conflict with the husband, multiple losses, the need to take control, and the difficulties in making a place for the new child. These women, like Hedda Gabler and Jeanne Hebuterne, were also struggling with financial problems created by pregnancy. The violence in the methods used seems to reflect the mother's need to take some definitive action in the face of these problems.

Pseudopregnancy

Barbara, at 20, had been married twice to the same man and once divorced from him. For several months she had been trying to live with him again. When he once again left her, she took several pills. In hospital she denied having overdosed and talked instead about her plans to join the army. However, her husband found a suicide note at home. She refused a pelvic examination, saying that her last period had been "on April Fool's Day." She left the hospital against advice before a pregnancy test returned negative. She had told her husband that she was pregnant. She described herself as a lifelong tomboy. She felt that her father had utterly rejected her after she had been forcibly raped at age 15. She had decided to abort an earlier pregnancy by her husband. That night, after leaving the hospital, Barbara shot herself with her husband's pistol while he was in another room. Autopsy revealed a lutein ovarian cyst, which may have caused the amenorrhea that she interpreted as pregnancy.

Late Pregnancy

Carol, 24, became pregnant with her third child several months after her husband's (incomplete) vasectomy. She had been depressed for several months because of the family's financial problems. When Carol was five months pregnant, she ingested a lethal dose of barbiturates but was resuscitated. She refused psychiatric consultation at that time. Two weeks before her expected date of delivery, she had an argument with her husband, and he took the children out. When he returned, he found her bedroom door barricaded from the inside (she had used her hope chest to bar the door). Carol was found dead of a barbiturate overdose. She had written the following note in lipstick on the mirror: "1. Cremated. 2. Bob and Ann only (her children). 3. Secret to everyone. Don't want to cause them humiliation. 4. Raised by husband. 5. All to kids. 6. Owe each $2000. 7. Education fund. 8. *They will be raised in California by me. Sell house and go out there.* 9. Bob and Ann to go to preschool and swimming. 10. Give them good birthdays and holidays and do things for them. I love Bob and Ann."

Postpartum

Maria, 25, returned for a postpartum check after delivering her second daughter. This pregnancy had been unplanned. Her husband was unemployed because of a back injury. Maria's older daughter had been a wanted child, born a year after the traumatic mid-trimester loss of Maria's first pregnancy. She and her husband had married during that first pregnancy. It was noted that Maria's grandmother and aunt were both dying of breast cancer and that Maria had overdosed with aspirin as a teen-ager. However, she seemed to do well during the pregnancy except for multiple minor physical complaints: joint pains, conjunctivitis, colds. She remained heavily involved in church work and said at the postpartum visit that she was "doing just fine." The next day, after an argument with her husband, she shot herself in the head in her kitchen while her husband and the children were in the next room.

The physical and relatively irreversible suicide methods chosen by these women bring into focus the need to identify and to treat such women before impulsive action preempts other solutions. All three of these women were under close medical supervision; still the suicides were not prevented. In retrospect, using even these fragmentary data, one can define certain warning signs: (1) a stormy marriage, (2) a history of a previous suicide attempt, (3) recent losses, and (4) evidence that the pregnancy has a negative rather than a positive value for the woman. Perhaps, had the Paris maternity clinic elicited this history from Jeanne Hebuterne, she would have been hospitalized. If there is in fact a continuum between peripartum suicide and child abuse/infanticide, obstetricians may need to learn from pediatricians the art of "hospitalization for social reasons." This could be as effective for pregnant women as for new mothers as a way to prevent the escalation of destructive impulses.

SECTION IV

PREGNANCY AS A PROTECTIVE OR PROVOKING FACTOR

Pregnancy as a protective or provoking factor in the causation of suicide in women of childbearing age has been the subject of recurring debate. The role of unwanted pregnancy as a possible provocation has long been suspected. It has been stated repeatedly throughout this book that completed suicide during pregnancy is a most uncommon event in recent times. In his chapter, Dr. Rosenberg demonstrates that pregnancy may, indeed, offer significant protection against completed suicide.

In an attempt to explain this protective mechanism, it is interesting to speculate that a biologic interrelationship may exist between a pregnant woman and her developing child which may foster a psychologic state which results in this protection. Dr. Marcel Heiman (1965) offered a psychoanalytic opinion on this phenomenon:

> *There are additional thoughts supporting the view that suicide during pregnancy may be less likely, without implying a reduction of the pregnant woman's suicidal potential. In depression, the aggression is turned against the self; this, however, follows the incorporation of the object representation. In the pregnancy of a depressed woman, a modification exists insofar as the fetus is identified (and/or fused) with the ambivalent or hated introjected object. Therefore the aggression does not need to be directed against the self, but can be expressed toward the fetus. May this result in such vicissitudes as abortion, premature labor, or stillbirth? After childbirth the aggression will be turned against the new object, the infant, still the representative of the incorporated hated object, or against the self, leading either to infanticide or suicide.*

This quote, as well as the opinion of others, leaves us with an overall impression that suicide in pregnancy is not a serious factor in mentally healthy women, but it should be carefully evaluated in those women with a preexisting or current psychiatric problem. Dr. Heiman's view could also be part of the explanation of suicide associated with pregnancy occurring predominantly in the puerperium.

Hormonal influences may offer another possible explanation for the protective role of pregnancy. High levels of estrogen during pregnancy seem to be associated with relatively higher levels of catecholamines. Since catecholamine deficiency may be implicated in the causation of depression, elevations of these hormones may tend to play a protective role during pregnancy. Their sudden drop in concentration after delivery may also be implicated in the increased frequency of various degrees of postpartum depression (Saks, Chapter 13). Current research on the relationship between catecholamines and human behavior in general may offer further explanation of these phenomena in the future.

Although these factors suggested that pregnancy has a protective role, it has long been suspected that unwanted pregnancy was the ultimate provoking factor to suicide in some women. Until the 1970s, laws against interruption of pregnancy were in effect throughout most of the Western world. The only ways by which a woman could terminate an unwanted pregnancy were on the basis of life-threatening illness to the mother caused by or associated with the pregnancy or on psychiatric grounds. Special hospital boards composed primarily of psychiatrists and obstetrician/gynecologists met to determine whether medical or psychiatric indications existed. This so-called "therapeutic abortion" was allowed to be performed only if a severe threat to a woman's life could be demonstrated. Therefore, generations of psychiatrists and gynecologists, not infrequently, compromised themselves by stating that the woman was likely to commit suicide unless therapeutic abortion was allowed, because she had threatened to take her life. Therapeutic abortions were not available to the vast majority of women, especially the poor; in New York City, therapeutic abortions were permitted only in approximately 1/1000 live births. Most unwanted pregnancies were terminated illegally. The incidence of morbidity and mortality which resulted following a self-induced abortion or an attempt by an ill-equipped and untrained lay person was unconscionably high. That women are no longer dying from illegal abortions is attested to by the fact that, in the first year (1970) in which legal interruption of pregnancy was permitted in New York City, maternal mortality dropped by half (Jean Pakter, consultant for the Bureau of Maternity Service and Family Planning, New York City Department of Health, personal communication, 1972) and has remained low, despite the fact that one of two pregnancies are electively interrupted. Because of the frequent medical complications resulting from illegal abortion, and the awareness of these complications by women, it should be considered that having a so-called criminal abortion may have represented some form of attempted suicide.

A number of years have passed since the revision of abortion laws. Yet, unwanted pregnancy may once more become a reality for some women. Since the United States Supreme Court decision in 1973, abortion on demand has been available throughout the United States. Similarly, elective interruptions of pregnancy are now permitted in most European countries. It appears that abortion legislation is a sensitive barometer of political and ethical or even religious pressures of a given time. Liberalized abortion laws can be and are occasionally reversed, if not by direct legislation then by inserting difficulties to providers, reducing or limiting facilities where abortions can be performed, or by withdrawal of funds from public assistance agencies (Medicaid). Further pressures now exist to reverse the Supreme Court ruling which, although proposed by the "right-to-life" movements, also have a measure of public support and support from the president of the United States (Ronald Reagan). Such a reversal would be particularly difficult to accept for those who sincerely believe that it is the woman's right to choose to bear a child. Therefore, we thought it appropriate to renew the debate on unwanted pregnancy.

Most studies support the view that when a woman is refused an abortion, it is most unlikely that she will attempt or commit suicide as a result of this decision. Even so, there were some reports which included a small number of women for whom unwanted pregnancy appeared to be the ultimate provoking factor. In 1955, Ekblad interviewed 479 women who had obtained abortion on psychiatric grounds. When asked what they would have done were permission for abortion not obtained, 3% stated that they would have committed suicide. This is further supported by Chalupa and Zdímalová (1968) in a report from Czechoslovakia. Of 28 cases of suicide in pregnancy in a five-year period, two women committed suicide apparently directly as a result of refusal of permission for abortion by a governmental commission. The study by Anderson (1961) from the Manchester University Department of Psychiatry in England also deserves mention. The effects of therapeutic abortion and/or sterilization on psychiatric grounds were studied in a working-class population over a 10½-year period. Of the 124 women who were followed, 95 had been referred for opinion on termination. Suicidal threats were made by 33 women (over one third) and six made suicide attempts. Only one woman committed suicide, about a year after termination was refused, and it was considered that this woman should have been allowed abortion.

One should be cautious in implying threat of suicide as a possible indication for abortion in previously mentally healthy women, unless there is a current disturbance. As one of the more rational voices, as early as 1943 and again later in 1951, Binder stated that the granting of a therapeutic abortion on psychiatric grounds should be based on the finding that the pregnancy has given rise to a state of grave, chronic mental stress and that the woman is less able to cope with psychiatric stresses. In addition to the concept that refusal of permission for abortion might be a predisposing factor to suicide in unstable women, it should also be considered that recommendation for abortion might have the same effect.

It is evident from Dr. Höök's chapter that most women will not actually commit suicide in cases of unwanted pregnancy if permission for abortion is not given. Dr. Höök, who is a recognized authority on refused abortion, discusses it in detail in her chapter. Her work in this area has been frequently quoted and is considered a standard reference on the subject.

Teen-age pregnancy is rampant in the United States (When Children Bear Children, 1983). Dr. Gabrielson's chapter is particularly pertinent because it deals with one of the many negative effects of teen-age pregnancy. He was the first to draw attention to the possible association between teenage pregnancy and subsequent suicidal behavior.

CHAPTER 9

SUICIDE, PSYCHIATRISTS, AND THERAPEUTIC ABORTION

ALLAN J. ROSENBERG*

An uneasy equilibrium exists between the pressures for interruption of pregnancy and the traditional codes in opposition. This conflict is poignant and personal for both patient and physician in each case considered for therapeutic abortion.

In the larger context, therapeutic abortion is an instrument of the wish to interrupt pregnancy as against the forces—physical, social, and psychological—for continuation. The number of unwanted pregnancies is always a significant one, and a study of family planning in America has shown that 16% of the most recent pregnancies in married women are not wanted by the wife or husband (Freedman et al, 1959). The proportion of unwanted pregnancies rose rapidly with the number of children the couple had had, from 6% in the first pregnancy to 62% in the ninth.

The influences in favor of the interruption of pregnancy have inevitably grown stronger in industrialized societies and have gained great impetus in view of the widespread concern about the dangers of the population explosion. In addition, it may be pointed out that the many forces of egalitarianism in our society support the drift toward the reduction of family size. Relevant to the present issue are the improved status of women and the greater importance of women in an economic role outside the home. Also many birth control measures are unequally utilized according to class position. As a part of this trend, there are constant pressures toward liberalization of the laws concerning therapeutic abortion in California.

In the more narrow context, therapeutic abortion is a device used to interrupt pregnancy where the criteria conform to specific legal requirements, namely, where continuation of the pregnancy imposes a danger to the life of the mother, which is the criterion used in the law of California and a majority of other states. The discrepancy between California law and actual practice is well established (Packard and Gampell, 1959). In a recent session of the California legislature, bills (Assembly Bills No. 2614 and No. 2310, 1961) were introduced to change the criteria from

*Originally published with Emmanuel Silver (deceased).

danger to the life of the mother to danger to the life or health of the mother and consideration of the soundness of the child.

If therapeutic abortion is considered as one element in the attempt to control the number of births or to forestall the possibility of unwanted children, then it is understandable that psychiatrists become involved in part because of their concern about rights and dignity (Szasz, 1960) of particular individuals with whom they deal and also because of their participation in efforts toward benevolent social change. In this communication we are concerned only with the psychiatric aspects of therapeutic abortion. Indeed, therapeutic abortion is now sought more and more frequently on psychiatric grounds.

The present study arose over the concern about the lack of systematic follow-up on women who had been evaluated for consideration of therapeutic abortion (on psychiatric grounds) and who were or were not recommended for abortion and were or were not aborted. It appeared that many psychiatrists were uncomfortable with the task of deciding whether or not the patient should be aborted if she came recognizably close to fulfilling the legal criteria; a number of psychiatrists did feel strongly enough about the matter to avoid getting involved in any way in this kind of determination. Further, it was observed that there were numerous inconsistencies in the attitudes and practices of psychiatrists who rendered these judgments, as evidenced by the presentations before therapeutic abortion committees on which the authors have served. The principal criterion for psychiatric recommendation is the likelihood of suicide as a danger to the life of the mother. The difficulty of this decision accounts in part for the lack of clear and consistent standards.

In order to clarify these issues, it was decided to embark on a pilot study to ascertain: (1) the availability of data concerning the attitudes and practices of psychiatrists who gave opinions regarding therapeutic abortion; (2) the availability of follow-up data on those women who had been considered affirmatively or negatively for therapeutic abortion (including those who were or were not aborted); and (3) the risk of suicide in pregnant women.

The findings seemed to be of sufficient interest and consistency to warrant reporting as preliminary results and to justify further investigation.

The California law makes abortion a felony "unless the same is necessary to preserve her life . . ." (California Penal Code). Considerations of the health of the mother or of the fetus are immaterial from a legal point of view.

PSYCHIATRIC PRACTICES

A questionnaire designed to elicit attitudes and practices concerning psychiatric indications for therapeutic abortion was sent to 100 psychiatrists, taken at random, in private practice in northern California. Sixty-nine responded.

The most striking feature of the answers was the lack of unanimity in the attitudes and practices of psychiatrists in a matter which is assumed to have scientific criteria and legal validity. For instance, one question had to do with the opinion as to the effects of pregnancy on mental illness. Fifteen of the respondents stated that morbidity was increased, 13 felt that pregnancy imposed relatively minor stress, and 25 were equivocal or indefinite in their opinions.* In a question designed to elicit the attitudes of psychiatrists toward doing such consultations, the split was almost down the middle, with 28 disliking doing them, 29 having little or no objection, and 12 not replying. Those who did more consultations reported less dislike of doing them and also tended to recommend abortion more frequently—a reasonably expected phenomenon. The range in number of such consultations done varied from a maximum of approximately 12 per year down to none. Further examination of the data showed that one group of five psychiatrists did about 35% of the reported consultations; the remainder of the 69 seemed to form another distinct group where there was a regular distribution over a range from three who did five to eight a year, to 18 who did less than one a year.

Of the 69 replying, 20 said that they had not treated or seen genuine suicidal attempts or psychotic reactions (no distinction was made between these two in the questionnaire) in pregnant women. However, 41 replied affirmatively, while four were equivocal and four did not answer. One question inquired as to whether it was improper or inconsistent for a therapist of a given patient to recommend abortion. Five respondents did not answer, 18 felt it was improper and, surprisingly, 36 felt that there was no impropriety involved. Ten gave equivocal responses.

In determining what the psychiatrists felt should be the criteria for abortion, it was found that virtually all respondents reported that suicide potential and psychosis were positive indications for recommendation. Also, a major proportion felt that a history of severe postpartum or severe antecedent mental illness should be among the criteria.

The opinion that the present laws are inadequate was virtually unanimous, and a wide variety of recommendations for change was suggested. A substantial number felt that socioeconomic factors, rape, incest, and extreme youth were factors which should be considered. Other indications suggested by a few were psychosis of the father, congenital diseases, problems of health and fitness and age of the mother or father, unwillingness to have children, divorce after conception, adultery, and narcotic addiction.

---

*Some responses may not total 69 since some of the questions were not answered by all respondents.

The data reported would seem to reflect the role of the psychiatrist in aligning himself with so-called progressive social change, particularly in these spheres where he can show concern for the welfare and dignity of the individual as a patient or as a member of society.

ATTITUDES OF PATIENTS

In an effort to determine whether it is possible to obtain follow-up data on patients, a questionnaire designed to elicit directly from the patient her attitudes about therapeutic abortion was sent to the 23 patients seen in consultation by one of the authors (A.J.R.) between 1952 and 1963. Of the 23, seven were not located, eight evidently received questionnaires but did not return them, and eight returned completed questionnaires. Those that were returned gave the distinct impression of being thoughtful, articulate, and detailed responses. Of the eight women who completed the questionnaires, three had received therapeutic abortions and five had not. While the numbers are not sufficient to form any substantial conclusions, the impression was conveyed that the patients generally seemed to be managing after the pregnancy, regardless of the outcome, much as they had before the pregnancy: the badly adjusted still having trouble, the more well-adjusted having less difficulty. These findings suggest that follow-up data on such patients are readily obtainable and systematic studies are therefore possible with larger numbers of patients, especially where there has been personal contact with the investigators. Arranging for follow-ups before an abortion is performed would undoubtedly facilitate these procedures.

RISK OF SUICIDE

It has been pointed out that the major criterion for the recommendation of therapeutic abortion is the risk of suicide.

Available evidence is equivocal. Swedish studies showed 8% of women who killed themselves were pregnant (Bengtsson, 1947). On the other hand, no suicides occurred among several large groups of women who were denied therapeutic abortion (Lindberg, 1948, SOU 1953/29). Observations in New York City (C.M. McLane, written communication, November 10, 1964; L. Weiner, written communication, November 24, 1964) suggest that proportionately fewer pregnant women commit suicide than those who are not pregnant. An attempt was made to evaluate this risk in California. Accordingly, coroners' records of three counties in northern California (San Mateo, Santa Clara, San Francisco), having a total population of about two million, were reviewed for the years 1961, 1962, and 1963. For this period, three instances of suicide by pregnant women were found. This figure was compared with the statistically predicted figure for women of childbearing age in the three counties. From this it was determined that the actuarial "expectancy" of suicides for the group involved was 17.6, in contrast to the three found in which the woman was pregnant.

These figures were arrived at in the following fashion. It was found that there was a total of 207 suicides in the three counties in the three-year period for women in the age span 16–50 years. The small number of three suicides in pregnant women seemed a noteworthy item, even though precise statistical analysis is not possible at this time. The comparable figure for the predicted rate has many variables relating to age groups, marital status, and correct reporting of suicides. The rough figure of a predicted number of 17.6 was arrived at by a comparison of the actual amount of time that any given woman of childbearing age is in a state of pregnancy as compared against the total childbearing period.

The algebraic computation was as follows:

$$\frac{T \times 36 \text{ months}}{P \times 9 \text{ months}} = \frac{207}{x}$$

(T represents the total female population of childbearing age, and P represents the total live births.*) Inasmuch as 207 represents the total number of suicides (age 16–50), x yields the predicted number of suicides for the pregnant population. The resulting figure of 17.6 is a minimal figure (it is based on the live birth rate and does not take into account pregnancies resulting in stillbirths and interruptions from other causes), and it therefore decreases the discrepancy between actual and predicted rates. However, as against minimization on this account, the standard for the total suicides introduces error of an indeterminate nature in that the childbearing age has been extended to 50. On the one hand, this would tend to increase the discrepancy because childbearing occurs more frequently in the lower periods of this span of years, but there is also some countervailing tendency in that the assigned childbearing period represents a smaller proportion of the total span. In summary, precise validation requires a finer statistical analysis, including division of women in the childbearing age into married and unmarried groups, but the number of actual suicides seems to be clearly less than expected.

The details about the cases of suicide were meager and fragmentary inasmuch as they were obtained from the abbreviated coroners' records. However, they seemed to be sufficiently interesting to warrant description even though significant conclusions cannot be drawn from so few cases. In one case a 25-year-old unmarried pregnant woman, living alone, shot her rejecting lover and then killed herself. Another case was a

*T was 380,905, and P was 129,408.

33-year-old multiparous wife of a serviceman: in the second trimester of her pregnancy she leaped from the Golden Gate Bridge. This woman was living on a military installation and in theory had access to medical care at no cost, and yet her depression did not cause those close to her to provide psychiatric care. It was said that the ostensible reason for her depressed state was her concern about the impending separation from her husband who was about to be shipped overseas. The third case was that of a 17-year-old woman who in the last month of pregnancy jumped off a highway overpass. The scanty data disclosed that she had recently come to California, having separated from her family of origin in Hawaii, and was in an environment of some stress and rejection in her new living arrangements with her husband's family.

DISCUSSION AND CONCLUSIONS

The data obtained from the results of the questionnaires returned by psychiatrists indicate a marked lack of consistency and uniformity in the attitudes and practices of the psychiatrists who are called upon to give opinions concerning psychiatric indications for therapeutic abortion. It would appear from the good percentage of response to the questionnaire and the free expression of opinion contained therein that the survey represents an accurate appraisal of the prevailing psychiatric viewpoints. From this, it can be inferred that the question of performance of therapeutic abortion is, to a large measure, dependent upon the particular psychiatrist who gives the judgment, and it becomes general knowledge as to which psychiatrist in a community is more liberal in his recommendations.

The extreme range of opinion represented among the psychiatrists is a far cry from the scientific objectivity that one hopes would apply to determinations affecting the life and health of patients. The range was from those who essentially never recommend therapeutic abortion to those who seem always to do so, from those who regard pregnancy as definitely increasing the incidence of mental illness to those who feel that pregnancy represents virtually no additional stress. While a fair preponderance of respondents reported having seen or treated severe reactions in the presence of pregnancy, this is not consistent with the small incidence of successful suicide recorded. It might be countered that more suicides would have occurred except for prompt psychiatric intervention or treatment in the form of therapeutic abortion; but it has also been observed that of the many women considered for therapeutic abortion, whether in fact aborted or not, very few seemed to proceed with any psychiatric treatment (Bolter, 1962). Further, the therapeutic abortions were done disproportionately more often in the limited number of patients belonging to the higher socioeconomic groups (Gebhard et al, 1958), so that this would, on a statistical basis, cast some doubt on the effectiveness of therapeutic abortion in preventing suicides.

The law at present deals only with the danger to the life of the mother. Should the law be amended at some future time to take into account the issue of danger to the health as well, then it would become necessary to assess the psychiatric morbidity, the incidence of psychosis during pregnancy, and postpartum psychosis in assessing the danger to the health of the mother.

It has been observed (Bolter, 1962) that the psychiatrist may be manipulated into distortion and exaggeration of the patient's disturbance, with the consequence that the clinical situation comes to approximate the requirements of the law in order to obtain the abortion desired by the patient or her physician. In some instances, iatrogenic pressures intensify symptoms so that discontent becomes illness. It might be pointed out about the issue of therapeutic abortion that it is one of the few entities in psychiatric practice in which psychiatrists readily take on the role of dealing with a symptom and the management of a symptom as a primary maneuver. This is highly contrary to the general current in psychiatric principles, and it directly conflicts with trends toward giving greater freedom to patients in their movements and decisions. For instance, in the management of suicidal patients, the tendency is to assume a substantial amount of risk rather than to attempt to guarantee absolutely against mishap.

One can only speculate that the willingness of psychiatrists to inject themselves into the role of decision-making about therapeutic abortion reflects some covert need. Superficially, it may perhaps represent some bending to the conscious wishes of patients and referring physicians, but one cannot feel that this is the only significant item. Perhaps it is more likely to be a projection of the psychiatrist's concern with the rights and dignity of the patient and the inadequacy of the present law.

The finding that the number of actual suicides was much less than the predicted number was surprising. Can it be assumed from this that pregnancy is a period of lessened vulnerability to stress rather than of increased vulnerability? If this is so, the reasons invite speculation. Perhaps physiologic and instinctive factors manifest themselves in greater maternal protectiveness. On the other hand, there may be effective mechanisms of increased social protectiveness and support. The fragmentary data about the three actual cases of suicide support a contention that the pregnant woman is less vulnerable because she receives greater social protection. In the cases cited, rejection, separation, and loss of support seem to be paramount. These factors appeared to be acute rather than chronic.

There are other implications. A pertinent one is that because of the lack of uniformity of psychiatric opinions, a case might be made for removing the decision entirely from the realm of psychiatric indications. If the social forces which manipulate psychiatrists into taking over this role are of sufficient strength, then perhaps this represents a trend which will be manifested by other developments. These could include translating the social needs by legislative procedure into consideration of the health of the mother as well as the (at present) exclusive consideration of life. A variety of other issues—social, medical, and psychologic—might merit scrutiny, such as the intactness of the fetus, economic status, extreme youth, illegitimacy, rape, incest, broken family, and the like. One might speculate further that the pressures toward facilitating the interruption of pregnancy could lead to removal of the decision from purely medical hands into a more representative body of opinion from the community at large, including others beside physicians. This would approximate the situation as it is at present in Denmark (1965). From the point of view of psychiatrists, such a change might be welcome in that psychiatrists seem to be forced into the position of making decisions which are basically nonscientific and, in fact, often contrary to the spirit of other trends in psychiatry.

It must be emphasized that the data reported here are preliminary and serve only to identify trends. These trends should be further tested and evaluated with larger numbers of patients since data seem readily available. Patients in this study were generally cooperative and willing to give information; any reluctance of physicians to approach them directly seemed unwarranted.

SUMMARY

Pressures for interruption of pregnancy by therapeutic abortion constantly increase, both for liberalization of laws and for interpreting existing law more broadly.

There are wide variations and inconsistencies in psychiatric attitudes and practices about therapeutic abortion. Follow-up patient data are scant, but necessary. Results of questionnaires indicate that such data can be obtained and convey the impression that patients seem to manage after pregnancy, regardless of outcome, much as they had before pregnancy.

This study indicates that the incidence of suicide in pregnant women is approximately one sixth that of the rate for nonpregnant women in comparable age groups, implying that perhaps pregnancy has a psychically protective role.

ACKNOWLEDGMENTS

Theodore A. Montgomery, MD, Department of Public Health, State of California, and Lincoln E. Moses, PhD, Department of Biostatistics, Stanford University, provided statistical information and consultation.

CHAPTER 10

SUICIDAL BEHAVIOR IN UNWANTED PREGNANCY

KERSTIN HÖÖK

Säv säv susa
våg våg slå
Sägen mig ver Ingalill
den unga månde gå

Fröding*

In poetry and fiction, self-inflicted death because of unhappy love is a recurrent theme. Infanticide has been used in many cultures to do away with malformed or undeveloped infants. In times of peril and starvation, the infants were the first to be sacrificed, perhaps with the exception of the first-born son.

The attitude to an unwanted pregnancy has shown considerable variation in different countries and in different societies. With the development of general hygiene, medical care, and obstetric progress, the chances for mother and children to survive childbirth and childhood have increased immensely in the past century. The population of the earth has reached such numbers that survival is again being discussed. A decrease in reproduction rate has become a worldwide urge and has led to the development of several contraceptive devices. Yet, for many women, secure and harmless methods are not available.

The reaction of a woman to an unwanted pregnancy has long been known to imply a risk for her life and health. Accordingly, the reactions of the society have aimed at preventing such unwanted pregnancy, or to ensure the health of the woman or of the fetus when the pregnancy is a fact.

Violent actions to solve emotional or cultural distress are still common. Suicide in unwanted pregnancy is known to occur. Suicidal behavior in unwanted pregnancy can be examined from many angles; some studies are directed to the various actions to which a woman may resort

Sigh, Sigh, Sedges in Guitar and Concertina: A Century of Poems by Gustave Fröding. Translated in the original meters by C.D. Locock. London, George Allen and Unwin, Ltd, 1925, p 80. Entire poem, translated in English, at end of chapter.

in an unwanted pregnancy, among which suicide or attempted suicide must be considered.

A number of studies have been directed towards the occurrence of pregnancies in women who make suicidal attempts. Several studies have pointed to the fact that attempted suicide may be just as common in pregnant women as among nonpregnant women within the same age group (Whitlock and Edwards, 1968).

In Sweden the suicide rate for women over 15 years of age is 0.1‰ (ie, 1:10,000). The rate is somewhat lower for young women 15–24 years of age, and it is higher in the age groups above 45 years of age (Sveriges officiella statistik, 1981.) This seems to be true also for the other Nordic countries.

The occurrence of suicide in pregnant women has, in recent years, been very rare in Sweden, which must be interpreted as being due to the fact that in cases of deep depression or suicidal threats the woman is given medical attention (Sveriges officiella statistik, 1978). If the pregnancy is unwanted and she applies for abortion, revealing suicidal threats, her application is probably granted.

From the official statistics in Sweden, it is found that during the period 1938–1958 three cases of suicide were registered following a rejection of an application for abortion. The 1965 enquiry committee on abortion (SOU 1971/58) made a survey of 18,618 applications for abortion to the Swedish National Board of Health in the years 1964–1966 and found four cases of suicide recorded for women who had had their applications granted. The suicides occurred before the abortion operations were performed. For the years after 1966, no suicides in women wanting abortion are reported.

Ettlinger (1975), in her careful evaluation of suicide prevention after attempted suicide, found that of 274 women only five (1.8%) were pregnant at the time of the attempt.

Otto (1965, 1971, 1972, 1982) has studied suicide attempts among young people. In records of 1376 girls under 21 years of age, 78 (5.7%) were recorded as pregnant. This frequency is comparable to figures by Whitlock and Edwards (1968); 7.2% of all women aged 45 years or less who made suicide attempts were pregnant.

In the Vienna part (Dr. H. Katschnig) of the World Health Organization study, *Suicide and Attempted Suicide* (1974), the subjects in the study were divided into two groups according to whether they confessed to being influenced by unhappiness motives, such as loneliness, loss of a dear one, etc, or by conflict motives in which other people were involved. Conflict motives were found in 70% of women of all ages, and unhappiness motives in 30%. In the age groups under 30 years of age, the conflict motives were even more frequent: six times more frequent than unhappiness motives.

Several of these studies stress the fact that, in follow-up studies of persons who have made suicide attempts, there is a considerable risk that the person will die in a later suicidal act.

Otto (1965, 1971, 1972a, 1982), in several papers, has presented his studies on suicide attempts in young people under 21 (25) years of age. He noted that the risk of repeated attempts of suicide is very great among young people who have once attempted to commit suicide. In his material, 11% of the boys died in the follow-up period of 10–15 years compared with 2% of the controls. Among the girls, 4% of these patients died compared with 2% in the control group. The majority of the dead children in his study had committed suicide. This was especially true of the boys and girls who had used active methods. There seems to be a maximum risk in the two years following the suicide attempt. Otto stresses the necessity of keeping in continuous contact with the patient during the time immediately following the attempt.

In Otto's (1965) study of 1376 girls who had made a suicide attempt, 78 were recorded as pregnant. The youngest of the pregnant girls was 14 years old. Otherwise, the age distribution was the same as that found for the nonpregnant girls. The majority of the girls belonged to social group 3.* There was no difference between the pregnant and the nonpregnant group of girls. Of the pregnant girls, 16.7% indicated that they had attempted suicide before; at that time they had not been pregnant. The majority of the pregnant girls mentioned the pregnancy as the provoking element for the suicidal act. Love problems were given as a cause in 65% of the pregnant girls and 42% in the nonpregnant.

Psychiatric symptoms were indicated in 28 of the cases where pregnancy was recorded. The majority of these pregnant girls showed neurotic depression (75%) or neuroses (17%). The nonpregnant women showed neurotic depression reactions in 27% and neuroses in 26%. Psychosis was seen in 15% in the nonpregnant and in none of the pregnant women.

Otto points out that an insecure or troubled relationship with a male partner presumably contributes to the desperate measures taken by the woman. The most critical time for a suicide attempt in pregnant women was the second or third month (19% and 23%, respectively), the period when the pregnancy is usually discovered.

In the studies that preceded the Swedish Abortion Act of 1938, there was much discussion on the risk of mental impairment during pregnancy and after delivery. Many authors mentioned the common occurrence of depressions during the first three to four months of pregnancy, stating that depression might occur even if the child was wanted and the social conditions for the woman were good. The term, physiological

*Lower socioeconomic group.

depression, has been used for this condition, and it is most common during the first three to four months of pregnancy (SOU 1964/40). Bertelsen et al (1977) found that in nine of 11 pairs of concordant twins with unipolar affective disorder, the depressive episodes were related to pregnancy or childbirth. In unfavorable situations, especially when the pregnancy is unwanted and the conflicts with the father of the child are severe or support by the woman's family is otherwise lacking, the depression can be very deep and give rise to actions of despair. Suicidal thoughts, and even attempts, are not infrequent.

A number of studies have started from the unwanted pregnancy, to evaluate its effect on the mother; some investigations have also aimed at evaluating the effect on a child born after an unwanted pregnancy (Höök, 1963, 1971, 1975; Matějček et al, 1978).

Deliberate termination of pregnancy is used by both primitive and advanced societies as a method to cope with unwanted pregnancy. In Sweden, this has been prohibited by law since the 13th century. If the mother's life is at risk, or in order to avoid serious damage to her health, an induced abortion would, however, not be punishable. The conflicts of interest arising in these cases nullify the criminal nature of the abortion.

SWEDISH ABORTION ACTS

The rules for performing induced abortion have been regulated in Sweden by the Abortion Acts of 1938, 1941, 1942, and 1946. The Swedish law of 1946 on therapeutic abortion stated that pregnancy may be terminated by legal abortion because of: (1) illness, physical defect, or weakness in the woman, when the birth of the child or the care of it might seriously endanger the woman's life or health; (2) when the woman has been made pregnant under conditions stated in the penal code, which have involved gross disregard of the woman's freedom of action (rape); and (3) when the woman or the father of the child might transmit a serious mental or physical defect or disease.

The acts of 1938–1946 were much discussed and prompted a number of studies on the effects of unwanted pregnancies in women when legal abortion had been applied for and it had either been granted or refused.

These investigations and the study by the 1965 Committee on Abortion (SOU 1971/58) have formed the basis for the present Abortion Act of 1974 (Socialstyrelsen, 1974).

1. Pregnancy shall be interrupted on the woman's request before the 12th week of pregnancy, unless the interruption because of illness in the woman is likely to impend serious risk to her life or health.

2. If the pregnancy is further advanced than 12 weeks, pregnancy can be interrupted on the request of the woman if special investigation has shown that there is no such risk as in 1.

3. After the 18th week of pregnancy an abortion is only granted for special reasons, and after the consent of the National Board of Health and Welfare.

STUDIES OF UNWANTED PREGNANCY

In Sweden, Ekblad (1955) made a comprehensive review of the literature. The material in Ekblad's study consisted of 479 Stockholm women who had undergone therapeutic abortion. These women were examined both at the time of the operation and at a personal follow-up examination 22–54 months later. The group was considered to be a representative sample of Stockholm women who are granted abortion for therapeutic reasons. In Ekblad's material, 3% of the women stated that they would have committed suicide if they had not been granted the desired abortion; 18% said they would have secured an illegal abortion.

Arén and Åmark (1957) carried out a follow-up examination in 195 women who were granted permission to have a legal abortion but did not undergo the intervention. They reported that one woman in their study had made an attempt to do away with herself after being refused permission for an abortion. After a second application her request was granted, but she eventually refrained from having the abortion performed. Two women in their study had later committed suicide, one and four years, respectively, after the application for abortion. Neither of them completed the pregnancy; both were married and in conflict with their husbands.

Hultin and Ottoson (1962) studied a group of 166 women who were referred by the National Board of Health to a psychiatric hospital department for clinical observation in connection with an application for legal abortion. In this material suicide threats had been made by about 50% of the women, or roughly twice as often as in a control series which had been selected from applicants for abortion of corresponding age, marital status, and domicile. The interpretation put upon this finding was that the threat to commit suicide had often been an indication for clinical observation in these women, whom the authors described as mentally frail individuals in an acute, alarming situation. No suicides occurred among these women.

The reactions of women whose applications for therapeutic abortion are refused were studied by Lindberg (1948). He investigated over a thousand women who had been admitted to a psychiatric clinic for an investigation as to a possible abortion. Of the investigated patients, 344 women who had been refused the desired permission for abortion constituted the group for the report. The author mentioned that in some cases it was necessary to give electroshock therapy to overcome the mental depression in the patient, whereas other women accepted their pregnancy fairly soon after their admission to the clinic. Some women, however, showed a violent reaction to the refusal and endeavored in various ways to demonstrate the difficulty of their situation. A threat of suicide was made by 18%. None of the 344 women actually committed suicide, however. The author considered that cases showing mental insufficiency of such severity that suicide really seemed imminent during the clinical observation had been granted the desired permission for therapeutic abortion.

THE AUTHOR'S STORY

The study group consisted of 294 women living in the Stockholm–Uppsala area in Sweden, who had applied to the National Board of Health to have a legal abortion and who had had their applications refused. A total of 484 applications of 4553 (11%) had been refused in the whole of Sweden during the same period (1948).

A search was made to ascertain the outcome of the pregnancy as well as the subsequent fate of the women and of the children in question. With the aid of census registers and parish records, information was obtained regarding the present place of residence and home address of all these women.

Seven women had left the country in the interval between the application for abortion and the follow-up examination. They could not be traced with complete certainty, nor examined, but from available information it seemed likely that the pregnancy in question had had very little to do with their wish to leave the country.

A group of 24 women who had been refused permission for therapeutic abortion differed from the others. Following the refusal of their original applications, these women had become worse, had applied again to the National Board of Health, and had then obtained the desired permission. As these cases are of interest from the point of view of their reactions during the period between the two applications, they will be discussed from this aspect.

Three women had died and therefore could not be examined. None of the deaths had any connection with the mental health of the women or with the pregnancy.

When the plan for the examinations was being drawn up, it seemed likely that the women might experience distress when they were reminded of earlier difficulties and emotional conflicts. However, with the aid of a social worker experienced in this field, it was possible for me to persuade 249 of 260 women (96%) to cooperate in a personal follow-up. In these women, full information regarding their reactions to the pregnancy in question and in the subsequent period could be obtained.

WOMEN WHO DID NOT WANT TO TAKE PART IN THE FOLLOW-UP EXAMINATION

A considerable amount of information on the subsequent fate and personality traits was also obtained regarding the 11 women who did not desire to take part in the investigation.

As a certain element of selection seems to be implied here, and as these women who refused to cooperate possibly had done so for reasons that might be of interest to an exhaustive follow-up study, a brief review of their reactions will be given here.

All the women who refused to cooperate had continued their pregnancies after their applications for therapeutic abortion had been rejected. One of them gave birth to a stillborn child at premature delivery and in two cases abortion with death of the fetus occurred in the seventh month. No information was obtained to indicate that the abortions had been induced. Three of the women had given the child away, and five took care of it themselves.

In eight of the 11 women in this group, evidence suggesting conflicts with the male partner or threats of social disgrace was present when they had applied for abortion. Five of the women had shown strong evidence of mental immaturity at the time of the application, and two others were diagnosed as having some other form of abnormal personality.

Also, the four women who were considered to have a normal personality possibly had reduced powers of coping with emotionally charged experiences. It would probably have been of value for the women in this group to have taken part in the follow-up examination, in spite of their fear and reluctance. The fact that in two cases the husband of the woman got in touch with the investigator, not only to supply information but also to seek advice personally concerning his wife's reactions, is evidence that the women were in need of external guidance in adjusting themselves to the emotions aroused by the rejected application for abortion.

SOCIAL AND CLINICAL STRUCTURE OF THE STUDY GROUP

Married women predominate among those who apply to the National Board of Health for a legal termination of pregnancy.

From the investigation carried out in connection with the application for abortion as well as from the information obtained at the follow-up, it was apparent that the occupation in question consisted of full-time or nearly full-time work (Table 10-1).

At the follow-up examination the women were questioned about the male partner; the examination was not extended to the man himself as he

Table 10-1
Occupation Outside Home and Marital Status at Application

	Married (%)	Divorced, Widowed (%)	Unmarried (%)	Whole Group (%)
Working	33	95	88	63
Not working	67	5	12	37
Total	100	100	100	100

was often no longer part of the woman's environment. Under these circumstances the data concerning the male partner must be regarded as incomplete; many of the women had subsequently had no further connections with him. The women's statements were checked as far as possible by a study of hospital records.

In a few instances, illness in the partner seems to have been the reason why an abortion was requested. Six percent of the partners were known to have been on sick leave for some bodily disease at the time of the application. Nervous disorders without concurrent alcoholism, causing incapacity for work, were reported in 8%. One man had subsequently been treated on repeated occasions for manic-depressive psychosis. Alcohol addiction without mention of primary mental disturbance, causing serious reduction in the power of earning a livelihood, was reported in 6% of the men. In 6% of the partners, penalties for unlawful actions were reported.

The distribution of the intellectual capacity did not show noteworthy differences from that found in a normal population.

PSYCHIATRIC DIAGNOSIS

It was found at the psychiatric exploration that many of the women had already shown signs of mental disturbance in some form, prior to the pregnancy in question. Only in a few cases, however, was endogenous psychosis suspected. These symptoms had already been considered in the medical report in connection with the application for legal abortion; either they had become accentuated during the pregnancy, or fears were expressed that the symptoms were progressing.

An attempt has therefore been made to give some psychiatric description of those studied, based on the documents filed for the abortion application, the findings at the follow-up examination, the anamnestic data given at the interview by the woman herself, and any other available documents and reports. In light of these findings, an evaluation of the occurrence of mental deviations in the women was attempted. For this purpose, the absence or occurrence of abnormal or deviant traits was registered. Any such classification is largely dependent on the training and subjective view of the individual investigator. The method of recording characteristics only on the basis of their presence or absence is rough; it is a question of an artificial dichotomy applied to continuous variables. The placing of a borderline between the presence or absence of negative traits in the personality is arbitrary. In the present investigation, the classification is based more on clinical common sense than on any particular psychiatric or psychologic theory.

If a woman had no noticeable deviant traits, she was classified as a normal personality. In the deviant personality group were placed women with obvious abnormal traits which either were observed at the follow-up or came out during the history-taking when the woman's tendency to display such characteristics during stress was mentioned.

It has often been stressed that the nature of symptoms has close association with the basic personality of the patient. It was found that the women in this study, when subjected to various kinds of stress, showed a form of reaction typical for each woman, regardless of the stressing factor. For the purpose of the clinical description, it was therefore decided to describe types of personality in which one particular feature is given a central position and other variables are ignored. The personality deviation was classified according to the most conspicuous symptom. Naturally, there was hardly a single one of these women who did not also display additional traits, but to introduce all personality traits that bordered on "abnormality" into the diagnosis would have required a much more comprehensive study than the present one to allow tenable conclusions to be drawn regarding the prognosis for the different diagnostic combination groups.

The types of psychoneurosis and personality deviations found in the material were grouped as follows:

Neurasthenia and psychasthenia Women with psychasthenic or neurasthenic traits were placed in one group, the major symptoms being fatigue, asthenia, and irritability, both mental and physical. Vegetative symptoms, such as headache, digestive disturbances, and insomnia were frequently found.

Anxiety neurosis and obsessive-compulsive states Women with anxiety neuroses were placed together with cases in which defense mechanisms in the form of phobias and compulsive actions formed the most conspicuous symptoms.

Depressive traits Women suffering from abnormally severe mental depression, lack of initiative, feelings of inadequacy and inferiority, often morning anxiety, were placed in this group.

Sensitive traits Women with heightened psychic vulnerability and a tendency to believe that the reaction of their environment was directed against themselves were characterized as sensitive cases.

Schizoid traits Women lacking in emotional warmth and with difficulties in making personal contacts were classified as schizoid in accordance with Kretschmer's (1951) definition. Bizarre ways of acting were noted in some cases.

Hysteroid traits The women belonging to this group showed marked affective immaturity and affective instability. In addition to displaying dramatic exaggerations, they lacked the capacity for insight into their own and other people's situations. In some cases the self-deception was extremely marked. The hysterical symptoms showed great variation. In the present study, there were no cases of conversion hysteria.

Immature personality Women of the type described as psychoinfantile by Lindberg (1950) were placed in a special group. This syndrome is characterized by desire for guidance and support and involves emotional immaturity, helplessness, and lack of self-confidence. It was, of course, natural that many of the younger women should display these mental traits at the time when they applied for abortion. Indeed, a striking feature among these young women was their lack of insight into the true implications of their situation—they looked upon the pregnancy as an exciting event and as a proof that they had become adults, but they had little understanding of the demands and problems that they would have to face. However, only those with persisting mental immaturity during the observation period and at the follow-up examinations were classified as having an immature personality in the present investigation.

Psychosis In a few women, the personality had become so distorted by psychosis that the prepsychotic personality could not be analyzed. These women have been placed in a separate group.

Table 10-2 shows the psychiatric diagnosis in relation to threats of suicide and illegal abortion for the 273 women studied.

RESULTS

In the primary group consisting of 294 women, no suicides occurred following rejection of the application for legal termination of the pregnancy. Neither were there any attempts at suicide, as far as can be judged from the information available.

In view of the absence of both suicide and attempted suicide despite suicidal threats, the implications of a threat to commit suicide might be interesting to study. Comparison with a threat to procure illegal abortion as another way out of a distressing situation was also considered important. These features were therefore investigated in the 273 women who were studied from this particular point of view.

Mental deviation had been noted in 16 of the 24 women who had the abortion accepted on a second application, but although abortion had been recommended in three cases of four at the first application, their

Table 10-2
Psychiatric Diagnosis and Threats of Suicide or Illegal Abortion in 273 Women

Psychiatric Diagnosis	Threat of Suicide	Threat of Suicide and Illegal Abortion	Threat of Illegal Abortion	No Threats	All Women
Normal personality	10	4	23	120	157
Deviant personality					
Neurasthenic and psychasthenic traits	1	2	7	20	30
Anxiety neurosis and obsessive-compulsive status	—	—	3	10	13
Depressive traits	1	—	1	6	8
Sensitive traits	—	—	—	3	3
Schizoid traits	—	3	5	3	11
Hysteroid traits	1	3	5	13	22
Immature personality	4	3	2	15	24
Psychosis	—	—	—	5	5
Total	17	15	46	195	273

symptoms at that time had not been considered severe enough for the desired abortion to be granted. At the second application, 20 women had expressed suicidal thoughts.

In this group of 273 women, suicide threats had been uttered by 32 of them (12%) and threats to secure illegal abortion by 61 (22%). A combined threat of suicide and illegal abortion occurred in 15 cases.

No connection was found between age and threats of criminal abortion or suicide. Furthermore, there seemed to be no connection between the fact of having already given birth to children and suicidal thoughts or threats to procure illegal abortion in connection with the present pregnancy.

It was also found that a threat to commit suicide occurred more frequently among women not married to the partner (25 of 157, 16%) than among those married to him (only 7 of 116, 6%). The difference is significant. A threat to procure illegal abortion did not seem to have any connection with marital status, however; instead, there was a significant connection between threats of criminal abortion and the emotional relations with the male partner at the time of the application. Forty-two (32%) of the 130 women who had been deserted by, or were in conflict with, the male partner threatened to procure illegal abortion, while only 19 (13%) of the 143 women with good relations with the partner expressed such thoughts. Threats of suicide, on the other hand, did not seem to have any connection with the emotional relations in this group.

Threats of suicide were expressed more often by women with a deviant personality (18 of 116, 16%) than by those judged to be normal (14 of 157, 9%); the difference is not significant, however. The same tendency was found with respect to threats to secure illegal abortion; 34 (29%) of deviant women and 27 (17%) of the normal women expressed such threats. The different diagnostic groups are small, however, and caution should be exercised in drawing conclusions. If each group is considered separately and compared with the others, it is found that suicide threats predominated significantly only among women with immature personality, whereas threats of illegal abortion predominated in women with schizoid traits.

DISCUSSION

The refusal of the abortion application thus seems to have brought forward thoughts of self-destruction. These thoughts were in many instances brought to the knowledge of the examining doctor by the relatives of the woman, not by the woman herself.

The threat to commit suicide might have been used to put pressure on the examiner, in other words it might have been an opportune threat. A more likely explanation, however, is that these women had, at the time of the examination, looked upon the unwanted pregnancy as a temporary condition, and it was not until after they had been refused permission for an abortion that the true gravity of the situation dawned upon them. Only then did they begin to realize the full implications for themselves and, faced with the responsibilities and extra strain that were now to be thrust upon them, they reacted with insufficiency symptoms characterized by desperation and lack of balance.

In all probability, those applicants for abortion who display personality traits or signs of mental illness of a nature suggesting an imminent risk of suicide are, in Sweden, primarily granted permisssion for a legal termination of the pregnancy and thus are never included in a study of rejected applicants.

The absence of suicide attempts among those rejected applicants in whom the investigating authorities had considered a definite risk of desperate actions to be at hand might be explained by the fact that the women had received a certain amount of support from their environment and possibly also because the desired therapeutic abortion had been granted after a renewed investigation.

Despite the absence of attempts at suicide in connection with their present pregnancy, seven women in the study are known to have attempted to commit suicide in other situations. Three of these had expressed suicidal thoughts in connection with the present pregnancy.

Two of the women who, after the renewed investigation, were given permission for a legal abortion had made suicide attempts in connection with family conflicts during earlier pregnancies; one of them was characterized as hysteroid, the other as immature. Attempts at suicide prior to the application had also been made by two other women, in both cases in connection with family conflicts; one was characterized as having a normal personality, and the other as hysteroid. Three women had attempted to commit suicide during the observation period.

In a study of young people who have taken an overdose of sedatives, Parker (1981) found that for the patients scoring low on the Beck suicidal intent scale, the overdose meant escape from tension, a kind of respite function, whereas on the same scale the patients with the high intent score perceived overdose and suicide in similar terms.

Kreitman et al (1969), in a study of attempted suicide in social networks, found that suicidal behavior is four times more common among friends and relatives of young people who have made suicide attempts than expected. He suggests that familial transmission of predisposition to suicidal behavior therefore more likely is culturally than genetically determined. The suicide attempt is a way of communication, a "cry for help."

Ettlinger (1975) states that the group of suicidal patients who are mentally ill show fewer suicides after support from the team in the prevention unit. Patients with emotional problems and family conflicts, however, do not seem to benefit from traditional psychiatric care. She suggests that psychotherapy, possibly including the family, would probably be more effective in bringing forth an element of hope for change.

A threat of suicide or an attempt at suicide, and in some cases even a threat to procure a criminal abortion in an unwanted pregnancy if permission for a legal abortion is refused, not only indicate a danger that the woman may expose herself to risks in connection with desperate actions, but may probably also be regarded as a sign of her inability to cope unaided with her situation. It would seem logical to interpret the connection between a suicide threat and difficult external conditions, such as not being married to the father of the expected child, and the occurrence of a threat of suicide particularly in a woman with an immature personality, as a plea to the environment for help and support in an intolerable situation, directed in the first place to the male partner or the parents and in the second place to the community as represented by the examining doctor and social worker. The implication of the suicide threat as a passive solution to a problem, or as evidence of an escape tendency, is in agreement with important personality traits in the immature woman.

The presumption that a threat to secure illegal abortion is an expression of more active tendencies in a woman is borne out by the fact that half of those who threatened actually did secure a criminal abortion. In all probability, such a threat is directed to the partner to a lesser degree than a threat to commit suicide. It is chiefly women who are in conflict with, or have been deserted by, the partner who talk of having recourse to criminal abortion; if the threat were actually put into effect, it would be more likely to loosen the ties with the partner and hence lessen the woman's possibilities for continuing the connection. Several of the women who terminated their pregnancy by unlawful means stated, in different connections, that they regarded the fetus and the pregnancy as an anomaly in their menstruation cycle which must be corrected as soon as possible; this was necessary for them as the condition constituted a serious threat to their security, a dangerous situation which presented insuperable problems of readjustment. This attitude, which was also seen in many of those who threatened to secure an abortion through illegal channels, is in line with the defective capacity for insight and compassion which are important schizoid traits; it may also be a sign of repression of unbearably distressing facts and experiences. The observation might be interpreted as indicating that women with such personality traits find difficulty in adequately expressing their feelings of incompetence at the prospect of continuing the pregnancy and taking on the responsibilities of motherhood, and hence their mental insufficiency is not judged to be serious enough to warrant a legal abortion.

Threats to commit suicide or to procure illegal abortion are therefore to be regarded both as symptoms reflecting the woman's feeling of insufficiency and incapacity at the prospect of handling the situation in which she finds herself and as an appeal for assistance.

The important measure that can be undertaken to help the patient is for the therapist to instill hope: hope for the future and hope that the conditions she finds unbearable can be changed.

SIGH, SIGH, SEDGES

Sigh, sigh, sedges,
Flow, waves, flow!
Now tell me of young Ingalill,
What way may she go?

Like the wing-shattered gull's was her cry as she sank in the mere:
'Twas when Spring was in green last year.

They were wroth with her, the good folk of Östanålid,
And it made her young heart bleed.

They were wroth with her, the neighbors, for her goods and her gold,
And the love that her heart did hold.

Stabbed with thorns in an eye's pure blue,
Black mud they cast on a lily's dew.

Then sing, oh sing your grief-song,
Ye little waves and low:
Sigh, sigh, sedges,
Flow, waves, flow!

CHAPTER 11

SUICIDE ATTEMPTS IN A POPULATION PREGNANT AS TEEN-AGERS

IRA W. GABRIELSON

Pregnancy, childbearing, and motherhood are normal biological events rather than disease processes, but even in the mature married woman they disturb the usual pattern of social life. For the teen-age girl, particularly if unmarried, pregnancy and the events which follow are especially likely to cause difficulty for the individual, those immediately associated with her, and society.

Other authors (Howard, 1968; Sarrel and Davis, 1966; Keeve, 1969) have reviewed some of the problems associated with teen-age pregnancies, such as disrupted education, welfare dependency, and increased fertility. A review of the medical records of 105 pregnant females 17 years of age or younger admitted to the Yale-New Haven Hospital for delivery during 1959 and 1960 suggested an additional potential difficulty—the possibility of suicide—threatened, attempted, or actually committed. This study revealed that 14 of the young mothers were known to have made subsequently one or more self-destructive attempts or threats serious enough to require care or to be reported to a physician at the hospital.

The study population received its obstetrical care in the period before the emphasis on programs for teen-age mothers. Some were patients of private physicians, but the majority were seen by obstetircal residents, medical students, and staff physicians in the general obstetrical clinic (Schleisinger et al, 1962). As a group they were offered no special social services, although in individual cases the need was so obvious that a social worker was assigned. They were excluded from school when their condition became apparent and limited educational alternatives were provided (Holmes et al, 1970).

Today in New Haven, and in many other cities throughout the United States, such girls are being offered programs that include unified medical care, augmented social services, and special educational provisions. It is hoped these programs will make a significant difference in the life of these young mothers and their children. Some reports are already indicating lower rates of medical complications among mothers and infants (Sarrel and Klerman, 1969) and decreases in early school terminations (Howard, 1968). Studies now under way may show that the attention being paid to the psychological aspects of pregnancy and the early childrearing period result in mothers better able to cope with the physical and emotional problems of their environment. If the programs are able to accomplish these goals, a marked reduction in the number of self-destructive attempts or threats would be expected. This paper hopes to assist those responsible for programs for pregnant teen-agers by alerting them to the need for listening for possible hints of future irrational acts and by stressing the urgency of long-term follow-up of this population. Research personnel may wish to use rate of suicide attempts as an additional measure of the success of special programs.

STUDY METHOD

The information about self-destructive attempts or threats was found in the course of a study concerned with intervals between conceptions in a teen-age population. The review of records was made at the Yale–New Haven Hospital in 1968, eight or nine years after the "index delivery" of 1959 or 1960. The group of 105 patients retained for study met the following three criteria: they were 17 years of age or younger and residents of New Haven at the time of the index delivery, and there was follow-up information available in the hospital chart for a period of at least two years thereafter. (Four exceptions were made to the latter criterion, where the records showed an additional pregnancy within a period of less than two years, although the follow-up stopped short of two years.) Such a review, limited to only one of the two area hospitals, and without a search of private physicians' records, certainly underestimates the number of suicide attempts and threats.

For the purpose of the hospital chart review, the following were classified as self-destructive acts: any self-mutilation such as wrist-slashing, jumping from buildings, the ingestion of any substance which the patient might have thought to be harmful, and the ingestion in obviously excessive amounts of any medication. In addition, two patients whose records showed a threat or fear of suicide were included in this group, hereafter referred to as the "suicide attempt" group.

The first section of this paper will describe the 14 patients in the "suicide attempt" group and the attempts themselves. In the following section, the entire population of 105 meeting the previously described criteria for inclusion in the study will be analyzed to determine which characteristics are associated with a higher risk of suicide attempt or threat. Finally, the rate of suicide attempts in this obstetrical population will be compared with the rates reported by others.

CHARACTERISTICS OF THE "SUICIDE ATTEMPT" GROUP

Selected characteristics of the 14 patients who made suicide attempts or threats are shown in Table 11-1. They ranged in ages from 13 to 17 at the time of their first 1959–1960 delivery. Eight were black, six white, and eight were Catholic, six Protestant. At the time of registration for care, nine were single and five had been married. The latter were all 17 and white Catholics. Only one patient had experienced a pregnancy prior to the one in 1959–1960.

By the time they made the suicide attempt, the patients ranged in age from 17 to 25. Eight were 17 or 18, one was 20, and five were 22–25. Eleven of the patients had been married by the time of the attempt, but four of these were already separated or divorced; three were still single.

In two cases the patient was pregnant with a second pregnancy at the time of the suicide attempt. For the remaining cases, the median number of months which had elapsed between the last delivery and the attempt was 20, with a range of 1–60 months. Four attempts were made in the first postpartum year and three of these were within four months of delivery. The median number of completed pregnancies at the time of the attempt was 2.*

Varied methods of suicide attempts were recorded. Ingestion was the most common. Five women had swallowed excess amounts of tranquilizers, sleeping pills, aspirin, or similar substances, and one claimed to have drunk ammonia. Four were treated for lacerated hands or wrists. One patient jumped from a third-story window, and another tried to cut herself with a razor and threatened to set fire to her clothing. In two cases, only a threat or fear of suicide was noted. In both there was also actual child abuse by the young mother or apprehension concerning infanticide.

Record review suggested that suicide attempts were often found in conjunction with the following:

Emotional illness Chronic psychiatric problems as well as acute episodes of depression or anxiety were noted in eight cases. Patients were described by terms such as ambulatory psychotic, depressed, disoriented, chronic anxiety, sociopath, and severe psychoneurosis. Patient 6 had an acute self-destructive psychotic episode requiring hospitalization. Patient 13 had "acute anxiety one month postpartum." Three patients—numbers 1, 8, and 14—had histories of previous suicide attempts. Patient 7 put her hand through a window on Christmas day, and patient 8 ingested aspirin on her 18th birthday. These latter two cases suggest the importance of situational stresses.

---

*In Connecticut it was illegal for physicians to prescribe contraception or counsel its use until June 1965 (General Statutes of Connecticut, Revision of 1958).

Table 11-1
Selected Characteristics of Patients Who Made Suicide Attempts or Threats

No.	Age at First 1959–1960 Delivery	Race	Religion	Marital Status at Registration	At Attempt: *Age*	At Attempt: *Marital Status*	At Attempt: *Completed Pregnancies*	At Attempt: *Months since Last Delivery*	Agent(s)	Other Significant Problems or Diagnoses
1	17	Black	Protestant	Single	20	Single	1	45	Wrist laceration	Two previous suicide attempts; termed "ambulatory psychotic" by psychiatrist—depressed, disoriented; pelvic inflammatory disease; much lung disease, lobectomy (1964)
2	15	Black	Catholic	Single	17	Single	2	20	Ammonia	Patient claimed she drank ammonia; examination was normal; returned to girls reformatory
3	15	Black	Protestant	Single	22	Separated	3	60	15 antihistamine tablets	Depressive reaction after marital separation
4	16	Black	Protestant	Single	23	Married	7	7	Sleeping pills	Pelvic inflammatory disease treated two days earlier
5	16	Black	Protestant	Single	17	Single	1	7 mo pregnant (2nd pregnancy)	12 Anacin tablets	
6	16	Black	Protestant	Single	18	Married	1	20	Attempted to slash self with razor and to set clothes on fire	Hospitalized in state mental hospital (1961); marital quarreling; pelvic inflammatory disease

7	13	Black	Catholic	Single	17	Married	3	31	Hand laceration	Put hand through window on Christmas day; marital discord; blunt affect
8	17	White	Catholic	Married	18	Married	1	3	10–15 aspirin tablets	Overdose of sleeping pills at age 14; took aspirin on 18th birthday after argument with husband
9	17	White	Catholic	Married	24	Separated	2	69	Wrist through window	Treated in psychiatric clinic for severe psychoneurosis related to broken marriage; pelvic inflammatory disease
10	17	Black	Protestant	Single	18	Married	2	4	Jumped 3 stories	Pelvic inflammatory disease
11	16	White	Catholic	Single	22	Separated	3	18	Tranquilizer	Treated in psychiatric clinic; husband and boyfriend narcotics addicts
12	17	White	Catholic	Married	25	Married	3	33	Laceration of wrists	Depressed; disoriented
13	17	White	Catholic	Married	17	Married	1	1	Threatened suicide and child abuse	Acute anxiety one month postpartum; infant found bloody
14	17	White	Catholic	Divorced	18	Divorced	1	5 mo pregnant (2nd pregnancy)	Fearful of suicide and infanticide	Previous suicide attempt with aspirin; hospitalized in state mental hospital for "nervous breakdown" (1958); seen frequently for anxiety

Marital discord Patient 3 ingested antihistamine pills "after marital separation." Patient 9 was seen repeatedly for psychoneurotic manifestations related to a broken marriage before being treated for a wrist laceration. Her husband "lives across the street with other women." Patients 6, 7, and 8 also had reported quarreling with their husbands.

Associated physical illness Five of the patients were seen for gonorrhea or pelvic inflammatory disease. Occasionally suicidal attempts occurred in close temporal relationship to treatment for one of these conditions. One patient suffered from chronic suppurative lung disease.

CHARACTERISTICS ASSOCIATED WITH RISK OF SUICIDE ATTEMPT

Table 11-2 analyzes the frequency of suicide attempts in the study population by selected characteristics.

Age The total study population ranged in age from 12 to 17 at the time of their first 1959–1960 delivery. Age at delivery did not appear to influence the risk of subsequent suicide attempt.

Race There was no appreciable difference in the risk of suicide attempt between the white and the black mothers.

Religion Twenty percent of the Catholic patients were in the suicide attempt group as opposed to only 9% of the Protestant patients. This excess risk of attempts among the Catholic mothers was found within each racial group, although the numbers were not large.

Marital status Subsequent suicide attempts were found in 22% of those mothers who were single at registration but in only 7% of those who were married at that time. One of the two who were separated or divorced at the index delivery made a suicide attempt.

When marital status was controlled for religion, there was a suggestion of independent association between each variable and suicide attempts. Being both Catholic and single was associated with approximately twice the risk found among those who were either Catholic or single. No suicide attempts were found among the married Protestants.

Residence The proportion of suicide attempts among mothers whose residence at the time of the index delivery was a nonpoverty area of New Haven (17%) was higher than the proportion of suicide attempts among mothers from poverty areas (11%).* Residence does not appear to alter the relationships found previously, ie, there was no difference in risk between racial groups within each of the two residential areas, but Catholics showed higher rates than Protestants within each.

---

*Defined as the lowest quartile nationally of the "Health Opportunity Index," developed by the Children's Bureau, based on the 1960 Census.

Table 11-2
Frequency of Suicide Attempts by Selected Characteristics

Item	Total Sample	Suicide Attempts	
		Number	*Percent*
Total	105	14	13.3
Age at delivery			
15 and under	22	3	13.6
16 and 17	83	11	13.3
Race			
Black	58	8	13.8
White	47	6	12.8
Religion			
Catholic	40	8	20.0
Protestant	65	6	9.2
Race and religion			
Black			
Catholic	4	2	50.0
Protestant	54	6	11.1
White			
Catholic	36	6	16.7
Protestant	11	0	0.0
Marital status at registration			
Married	62	4	6.5
Single	41	9	22.0
Separated or divorced	2	1	50.0
Marital status and religion			
Single			
Catholic	8	3	37.5
Protestant	33	6	18.2
Married			
Catholic	30	4	13.3
Protestant	32	0	0.0
Separated or divorced			
Catholic	2	1	50.0
Protestant	0	0	0.0
Residence at index delivery			
New Haven			
Poverty areas	64	7	10.9
Nonpoverty areas	41	7	17.1
Residence, race, and religion			
New Haven, poverty area			
Black			
Catholic	4	2	50.0
Protestant	37	3	8.1
White			
Catholic	19	2	10.5
Protestant	4	0	0.0

Table 11-2 (*continued*)

Item	Total Sample	Suicide Attempts *Number*	Suicide Attempts *Percent*
New Haven, nonpoverty area			
Black			
Catholic	0	0	0.0
Protestant	17	3	17.6
White			
Catholic	17	4	23.5
Protestant	7	0	0.0
Birthplace			
Connecticut	62	9	14.5
Other northern states	7	0	0.0
Southern states	34	5	14.7
Non-US or unknown	2	0	0.0
Source of care			
None	8	1	12.5
Clinic	79	10	12.7
Private	18	3	16.7
Outcome of delivery			
Full-term live birth	94	14	14.9
Premature live birth	9	0	0.0
Stillbirth	2	0	0.0
Parity			
No previous pregnancies	91	13	14.3
One or more previous pregnancies	14	1	7.1
Number of subsequent pregnancies (to date of last follow-up)			
None	8	2	25.0
1–2	45	7	15.6
3 or more	52	5	9.6
Complications of pregnancy			
No complications	29	0	0.0
Complication recorded	76	14	18.4
Venereal disease			
Reported	24	5	20.8
None reported	81	9	11.1

Birthplace There was no clear association between any particular area of birth and a higher or lower risk of subsequent suicide attempts.

Source of care The risk of suicide attempts was slightly higher among patients receiving prenatal care from private physicians than among those cared for in the hospital clinics or receiving no prenatal care at all. The numbers are too small to reach definite conclusions, but the trend is consistent with the finding of higher risk in pregnant girls from nonpoverty areas.

Outcome of index delivery All of the suicide attempts were among mothers who delivered full-term live babies. No attempts were recorded among those delivering stillborn or premature infants.

Parity Of the total population of 105, 91 were nulliparous at the index pregnancy and 14 were having a second or third child. There was no evidence that women of higher parity were at greater risk for subsequent suicide attempts.

Number of subsequent pregnancies There was a higher risk of suicide attempt among those women who had no more than two subsequent pregnancies during the study follow-up period (17%) as compared to those with three or more subsequent children (10%). Only eight of the total population had no pregnancy subsequent to the index pregnancy; of these, two attempted suicide.

Complications of pregnancy Seventy-two percent of the study population had complications, recorded in the hospital chart, with one or more of their pregnancies. These complications included such things as anemia, toxemia, infection, and hemorrhage. (Venereal disease was considered separately.) All 14 suicide attempts were among those who had complications recorded. None of the patients without complications were known to have made suicide attempts.

Venereal disease Almost one quarter of the study population had a diagnosis of venereal disease recorded in the chart at some time. Those with this diagnosis had approximately twice the risk of subsequent attempt (21% to 11%).

It is not possible to demonstrate statistical significance for the differences related to the above characteristics, primarily because of the small numbers involved. Chi-square tests show that only one of the above comparisons is significant at the conventional 5% probability level. Consequently the differences observed here are best regarded as suggestive leads. Further research may clarify the importance of the association of these factors with the risk of suicide attempts.

RELATION TO OTHER STUDIES OF ATTEMPTED SUICIDE

Before any conclusions can be drawn about the possible relationship between suicide attempts or threats and teen-age pregnancy, it is necessary to determine whether the frequency of attempts is higher in this sample than in the general population or in other adolescent groups. Although the incidence of suicide carried out to completion is relatively well known, at least for those cases reported to the medical examiner, few attempts have been made to develop directly an incidence rate of attempted suicide. Moreover, since previous studies have shown that major differences exist between individuals who make suicide attempts and those who actually commit suicide (Stengel and Cook, 1958; Shneidman and Farberow, 1961), extreme caution must be exercised in using suicide rates in connection with studies of attempts. An alternative method of deriving comparative figures is by using studies which have developed a ratio between attempted and completed suicide.

For the year 1957, Shneidman and Farberow (1961) collected information on completed suicides from the Los Angeles coroner's office and on attempts from the records of the Los Angeles County General Hospital, the 16 Los Angeles municipal emergency hospitals, and a questionnaire sent to all private physicians and osteopaths in the Los Angeles area. The hospitals reported 2019 attempts and the doctors an additional 3887, for a total of 5906. Since there were 768 completed suicides in the same period, the overall ratio between attempts and completed suicides was 7.69:1.*

Unfortunately, of those cases reported by doctors, data on only 633 were complete enough to analyze by demographic variables such as sex and age. Based on these incomplete data, the ratio of attempted to completed suicides for females of all ages was almost identical with the overall rate, 8:1; for males it was only 1.5:1. For both sexes at ages 10–19, the ratio of attempted to completed suicides was considerably higher: about 18:1. The difference between the sexes in this age group is especially striking: for males the ratio was about 5 or 6:1, but for females it was between 69 and 78:1.† For all ages combined, barbiturates and poisoning accounted for 52% of the female suicides and 63% of the attempts (for males the comparable percentages were 17% and 43%); no breakdown of method by age is given.

Working in New York City, where the reporting of accidental and intentional poisoning is mandatory under the city health code, Jacobziner (1965) developed a ratio of attempted to completed suicides based on reports of ingestion in the adolescent population. For the years 1960–1961, he found 568 attempted and five completed suicides by ingestion of chemical agents in the under-20 age group, yielding a ratio of over 100 attempts to one completed suicide.

Comparing the information from Jacobziner (1965) about attempts in 1960–1961 with his classification by sex and method of completed

---

*This figure is quite close to the less than 6:1 figure quoted by Stengel and Cook (1958), which they state is based on data from the police reports of Los Angeles and Detroit.

†These ratios were extrapolated from Shneidman and Farberow's tables in which entries are rounded to whole percentage points. The ratios which can be deduced from these data have the following ranges: for both sexes 18:1 to 19:1; for males 5:1 to 6:1; for females 69:1 to 78:1.

suicide in 1961–1962, the ratios for males and females were each found to be over 100:1. On the hypothesis that ingestion represents 50% of the attempts among female teen-agers (as was found in our sample), the ratio for all methods would be about 50:1.

The discrepancy between these two sets of ratios (based on Shneidman–Farberow and Jacobziner) can be partially explained by differences in the study populations and research designs. The Jacobziner study depended upon reporting, which is less complete in attempted than in committed suicides. Shneidman and Farberow, on the other hand, sought out the information, although their success with returns from doctors was not outstanding. The smaller size of the sample in the Jacobziner (1965) study also might result in greater variability. Sampling fluctuations and the rather crude methods used to produce comparable figures also may have contributed to discrepancies. Unfortunately, neither study provides the data necessary for a more accurate estimate, since Jacobziner (1965) does not deal with suicide attempts other than by chemical ingestion, and Shneidman and Farberow (1961) do not classify their population by both age and sex.

In the study reported in this paper, 105 patients were followed for a total of 7084 patient-months, or 590.3 patient-years. Thus there are about 590 "women years" of risk at average ages of 16–22 years. On the basis of the 12 mothers who made actual suicide attempts, this is a yearly rate of

$$\frac{12 \times 100}{590.3} = 2.03\%, \text{ or 2030 attempts per 100,000 per year.}$$

In order to determine whether this rate of suicide attempts was larger than that expected among young females in an urban population, the rates based upon the Shneidman–Farberow and Jacobziner studies were applied to suicide rates from Cook County, Illinois, in 1959–1963 (Maris, 1969) where the rate was 2.5/100,000 per year among females in the 15–24 age group. Applying this suicide rate to the estimated ratios of suicide attempts to suicides, one would expect between 173 and 195 suicide attempts per 100,000 per year using the ratios based upon Shneidman and Farberow's data, and 125 per 100,000 per year using the ratio based upon Jacobziner. The rate of suicide attempts in the study sample is roughly 10 times larger than the largest of these estimates.

DISCUSSION

At least two alternative explanations can be advanced to explain the major finding of this study: that the rate of attempted suicide among teen-age mothers is in excess of that which would be expected in the general urban adolescent population. The first explanation is that the stresses of pregnancy and child-rearing in some young girls are so enormous that they react by attempting suicide. An equally interesting possibility, however, is that the suicide attempt is not a direct result of the pregnancy, but that both the pregnancy and the suicide attempt stem from a common process. Both these events may represent disturbed behavior by adolescent girls. Girls who become pregnant in their teens may be demanding attention or trying to punish or inflict pain on their parents or other significant persons in their environment. Similarly, the suicidal act or threat may be a way of striking out or seeking revenge.

A study of suicide attempts in pregnant women by Whitlock and Edwards (1968) seems to support this latter alternative. They noted that the "majority of suicidal attempts by the pregnant women were impulsive, often precipitated by violent interpersonal disputes which did not necessarily relate to the pregnancy. The women showed marked instability of personality and many had experienced life-long interpersonal and sexual difficulties. A follow-up survey of two thirds of the patients showed that 37% of the women continued to show major psychiatric disorders."

Further research would be necessary to determine whether either of the alternative explanations offered would account for the increased rate of suicide attempts or threats in this population.

RISK OF SUICIDE ATTEMPT

The data reported earlier in this article on the association between specific characteristics and suicide attempts suggest that a higher-risk group might be defined within a population of teen-age mothers. The factors associated with an increased risk of suicide attempt within New Haven were: being Catholic, not having married, living in a nonpoverty area, experiencing a complication of pregnancy, and having a venereal disease at some time. The religion and marital status variables are especially notable since they run contrary to some studies of committed suicides. Since Durkheim's (1951) classic study, it has been assumed that committed suicides were lower among Catholics than other religious groups. Recently this conclusion has been questioned (Morphew, 1968). Relative to marital status, Seiden (1969) recently pointed out that, although suicide is less frequent among married persons, this is not true in the young married population. Under the age of 24, and especially under 20, the death rates from suicide were higher among married men and women than among single men and women. Seiden suggests that "perhaps youngsters who marry in their teens are seeking to escape from unsatisfactory home environments, or perhaps early marriage, per se, introduces stresses which lead to suicide."

The fact that women who were single, Catholic, and not living at a poverty level were more likely to attempt or threaten suicide than other women who also had borne children in their teens would seem to suggest that the acceptability of the pregnancy in the women's social group might be a contributing factor. Certainly in almost all groups, regardless of age, it is more acceptable to be pregnant if one is married than if one is not. Catholic religious training places strong proscriptions on sexual activity outside of marriage.* Finally, although teen-age pregnancies undoubtedly occur in large numbers in the middle and upper socioeconomic groups, in the public mind pregnancy at a young age is associated with illegitimacy and with the lower socioeconomic class. Therefore, when a teen-age girl who is single and/or Catholic and/or living above the poverty level finds herself pregnant, she may be more aware of the disapproval of her social group than she would be if she were a married and/or non-Catholic and/or a poverty-level teen-ager. This awareness of deviance from the norms of the group may make a suicide attempt or threat more likely.

Several of the findings indicate that those who attempt suicide represent a disturbed population: the high rate of venereal disease—which is often associated with promiscuity—and the frequent histories of emotional illness including psychiatric symptomatology, of previous suicide attempts, and of marital discord. Moreover, the high rate of pregnancy complications among those who threatened or attempted suicide, and the presence of physical illness in conjunction with several of the attempts suggest that physical conditions should not be overlooked. Venereal disease may be viewed as both an emotional and a physical factor.

SIGNIFICANCE OF THE SUICIDE ATTEMPT

Given what appears to be an excess number of suicide attempts among women who become pregnant in their teens, a question can be raised about the importance of this act. Is committed suicide a real possibility in this population? If it is not, is the suicidal behavior important in itself?

Several studies have shown a high rate of completed suicide among those who previously attempted or threatened suicide, ie, suicide attempters are a high-risk group for completed suicide (Shneidman and Farberow, 1956; Stengel, 1962). In addition, another study undertaken by the authors of this paper uncovered two apparent suicides in an obstetrical clinic population which delivered from 1963 through 1965. One

*Kinsey et al (1953) studied the association between religion and feelings of regret about premarital coitus among women. Although the differences were greater between the more or less devout within the religious groups, 35% of the devout Catholics as compared to 23% of the devout Protestant women regretted the experience.

took place two years after delivery but while the girl was pregnant with her third child; the other, three years postpartum. Pugh's (1963) analysis of mental disease related to childbearing is also relevant to this question. Considering first admissions to Massachusetts mental hospitals, he found a large excess of admissions with psychosis during the first three months postpartum for childbearing women as compared to nonchildbearing women. The risk of hospitalization was highest at the extremes of age, including the 15–19 age group. In a personal communication, Pugh noted that two of the 75 women in this childbearing group later committed suicide, eight months and one and a half years postpartum, respectively. These data suggest that although suicide carried to completion during pregnancy may be uncommon,* suicide is a significant risk in the postpartum period, particularly among those with a history of suicide attempts or of mental illness.

Even if completed suicide were not a significant risk, there would be important reasons to pay attention to the suicide attempt. First, physical harm to the woman or her infant is a frequent sequel of such attempts. Second, the attempt conveys a message to the environment. Rubenstein et al (1958) have suggested that a suicide attempt should be considered "not as an effort to die but, rather, as a communication to others in an effort to improve one's life." The message should not be ignored by the helping professions, even though it was originally directed to people important in the pregnant patient's life. The young woman who attempts or threatens suicide is consciously or unconsciously signaling to the world that she needs help. If this alarm is not heeded, there may be dire consequences for the individual and her child.

Siegal and Friedman (1955) have commented on the impact of suicide threats: "The threat of suicide forces people to marry, prevents marriage dissolution, coerces companionship between persons despite their mutual infidelity, prevents marriages, forces parents to acquiesce in their offspring's vicious habits, precludes institutionalization, is rewarded by escape from military service, is used to obtain favored treatment over siblings, is employed as a device to avoid military induction, etc." Stengel and Cook (1958) criticize the negative connotations of this list and point instead to the "frequency with which the suicidal attempt was found to have been the only effective alarm signal to mobilize long overdue medical and social help." They feel that suicide attempts consciously or unconsciously have important social effects, ie, they modify the human environment.

---

*Actually such suicides may not really be uncommon but merely underreported. Newspaper accounts of suicide pacts between unwed adolescent couples often cite pregnancy as a factor.

PREVENTION OF SUICIDE ATTEMPTS

Finally, what can be done to prevent suicide attempts or to help those who have made them? Unfortunately society has made little progress toward solving the problem of the disturbed adolescent. The education of parents and the creation of a healthy emotional climate would appear to be the first line of prevention. In addition, some program suggestions can be made. The tendency of physicians to treat a suicidal remark as a meaningless gesture should be modified. It may be only a gesture in the sense that suicide has a low probability of occurring, but it is not meaningless. It is an important sign and should be treated vigorously.

The multidisciplinary programs for teen-age mothers being developed across the country, with their concentration on individualized care for medical, educational, and social problems, should help detect patients at risk for suicidal acts, as well as provide the help which may make such a dramatic "alarm signal" unnecessary. It may be necessary, however, to mobilize additional psychiatric resources in order to provide individual and/or group therapy, not only for those who have already made a threat or attempt, but also for the high-risk group. Regardless of the reason for the suicide threat or attempt, the findings clearly indicate the need for increased concern with the psychological and emotional needs of the pregnant adolescent both during her pregnancy and for several years after delivery. They also suggest that the rate of suicide attempts may be another variable to study in the evaluation of special programs for this population.

SUMMARY

A review of the records of 105 New Haven residents who were 17 and under when they delivered an infant revealed that 14 had subsequently attempted or threatened suicide. Comparison with other studies indicates that the rate of attempted suicide in this population is higher than would be anticipated. Within the total study population, the risk of attempting suicide was somewhat higher among single girls, Catholics, and those not from poverty areas. Suicide attempts were also associated with pregnancy complications and venereal disease. It is suggested that this excess of suicide attempts may be due to the stress of the pregnancy or that both the pregnancy and the suicide attempt or threat may be forms of disturbed adolescent behavior.

The dangers of committed suicide or physical harm, and the "signal for help" function of the attempt, strongly suggest the need for preventive measures, including early detection and intensive treatment of long duration for both the suicide-prone and those who have threatened or attempted suicide.

ACKNOWLEDGMENTS

The study upon which this paper is based was supported by grants H-118 and H-231 C 1 and 2, Children's Bureau, DHEW.

This is a revised version of a paper presented before a Joint Session of the Maternal and Child Health, Health Officers, and School Health Sections of the American Public Health Association at the Ninety-Seventh Annual Meeting in Philadelphia, PA, November 10, 1969.

SECTION V

PSYCHIATRISTS' VIEW OF SUICIDAL ACTS DURING PREGNANCY AND THE PUERPERIUM

Dr. Rosenbaum's chapter gives an overview of the psychodynamics of pregnancy. The psychological changes and various moods associated with childbearing are discussed in an effort to understand suicidal behavior during pregnancy and the puerperium. Dr. Rosenbaum is a psychiatrist with particular interest in the psychology of women and their sexuality.

Postpartum depression and other psychotic diseases, rare as they may be, can emotionally overwhelm the recently delivered woman, sometimes culminating in suicidal behavior and even infanticide. The rarity of this condition may be, in part, due to the fact that unwanted or unplanned pregnancy is much less frequent in recent times. The lesser form of psychosis, postpartum depression, is also less frequently observed because the length of in-hospital stay for childbirth is only a few days in normal women.

Traditionally, it has been accepted obstetrical dogma that, however rare, attempted or completed suicide in association with pregnancy is most likely to occur during the postpartum period. It is particularly sobering, therefore, to consider Sim's (1963) observation from a study on the predictability of puerperal psychosis and suicide as an indication for abortion. He stated that of 213 women who were admitted to a psychiatric hospital in Birmingham, England, with a diagnosis of postpartum psychosis, none committed suicide. With the exception of Sim's data, most reports of postpartum mental illness include instances of suicide.

In her chapter, Dr. Saks discusses postpartum mental illness in some detail. Her initial training in obstetrics complemented her subsequent career training in psychiatry. This allowed her a unique opportunity to comment on the current thinking about the possible endocrine and neurochemical causes of postpartum depression.

Dr. Destounis' chapter describes postpartum psychiatric syndromes from a psychoanalytic approach aimed at prevention. He, too, has a long-time interest in the psychology of women, especially during pregnancy.

Dr. Astrachan also had training both in obstetrics and psychiatry. He discusses the subject of severe psychologic disorders of the puerperium, including attempted suicide, by stressing the clinical approach aimed at early recognition and prevention. He points to the need for greater interdisciplinary collaboration on these patients.

These pertinent articles on postpartum behavioral changes, concentrating on their association with suicide, have been included without any claim to a comprehensive discussion of postpartum depression.

CHAPTER 12

PSYCHOLOGICAL ISSUES IN PREGNANCY

MAJ-BRITT ROSENBAUM

When a pregnant teen-ager kills herself by stepping in front of a train, it makes news headlines (Darkness at Noon, 1983) precisely because it occurs so rarely. Gone are the days when one of the main reasons for legally terminating a pregnancy was the psychiatric assessment of high suicidal risk (Asch, 1965). Instead we are puzzled by the observation that suicide is less of a risk in pregnant women than in nonpregnant women (Sim, 1963, 1968; Otto, 1972). During the postpartum period, the risk for suicide increases and appears to be related to long-standing psychiatric problems (Report on Confidential Enquiries into Maternal Deaths in England and Wales 1973–1975). A parallel phenomenon is observed in regard to major psychiatric illness, eg, disorders of psychotic proportions, necessitating psychiatric hospitalization. The incidence of severe psychiatric illness is considerably lower during pregnancy than for a control population of women, but rises dramatically during the postpartum period, to two to four times the expected rate. During the past 100 years, there has been little change in the proportion of women suffering from postpartum psychotic illness; it is still estimated to be about one to two per 1000 (Kroger and Freed, 1951; Thomas and Gordon, 1959; Hamilton, 1962; Pugh et al, 1963; Kaij and Nilsson, 1972; Sandler, 1978). These postpartum psychoses are predominantly of an affective nature, with manic-depressive or depressive illness outweighing the schizophrenias (Donaldson, 1978; Kadrmas, 1979).

Based on these findings, it has long been customary to view pregnancy as an emotionally relatively calm period in a woman's life, a period that "since time immemorial has been considered the acme of feminine psychosexual development" and the fulfillment of "the ultimate feminine role" (Kroger and Freed, 1951). Most women today still consider pregnancy a time when deep and powerful wishes come to fruition, a time of creativity and self-realization (Nadelson, 1978; Brown, 1979). However, the increasing interest in studying the psychological life of the pregnant woman has served to highlight pregnancy as a time of considerable stress, a period that can challenge a woman's adaptational capacities to their limit. It is a time in her life when her coping skills often stretch to the breaking point, as she experiences psychiatric symptomatology in the form of anxiety, phobias, mood disorders, and obsessive-compulsive or psychosomatic concerns. In fact, there is an increasing body of evidence pointing to pregnancy as a period characterized by high levels of anxiety that finds its expression in many varieties of psychological symptoms (Grimm et al, 1967; Morris, 1968; Shereshefsky and Yarrow, 1973; Lubin et al, 1975; Hatherly et al, 1979). Thus, it has been an oversimplification to judge the psychological state of the pregnant woman on studies of severe psychopathology or on the clinical observation that some women with chronic or recurrent psychiatric illness can handle pregnancy well or even fare better during pregnancy than at other times (Sandler, 1978).

Statistically there appears to be a short period during pregnancy that may qualify as a calm, emotionally contented state, that is, mid-pregnancy—the 20th to 34th week, but only in relation to the other periods of pregnancy (Grimm, 1961; Shereshefsky and Yarrow, 1973; Brown, 1979). Previous anecdotal or clinical observations of the anxious state of the pregnant woman have recently been substantiated statistically. For instance, a prospective study from Sweden (Kaij and Nilsson, 1972) of 800 women followed throughout their perinatal period indicated that 17% had substantial neurotic reactions during pregnancy, rising to 19% postpartum; 27% had moderate neurotic symptomatology during pregnancy (27% postpartum), and only 16% were symptom-free during the pregnancy (28% postpartum). A study from Uganda of 119 pregnant women showed that the 6.7% rate of demonstrable psychopathology they exhibited prepregnancy rose to 17% during pregnancy, remaining at that level postpregnancy (Kumar and Robson, 1978). Other studies indicate that up to 84% of pregnant women suffer some degree of depression (Cohen, 1973).

The culturally idealized "mother myth," the social tolerance and support of the pregnant mother and of her needs and "unusual" wishes or whims, the biological protection offered by the changed physiology, and the altered psychodynamic state of the pregnant woman all contribute to the fact that we tend to ignore or minimize the psychopathology and the psychological stress to which pregnant women are subject. In this regard, it has been repeatedly noted that pregnant women are more "regressed" psychologically, more dependent, more in touch with their inner conflicted feelings, and more frequently aware of hostile, violent fantasies with vivid imagery of disaster, death, and murder (Bibring, 1959; Heiman, 1965; Colman, 1969, 1971; Benedek, 1970). They also report a high incidence of dreams of misfortune and harm, and threats of destruction of the self or the baby (Wilson, 1968; Shereshefsky and Yarrow, 1973). In my practice I have been struck by how frequently both homicidal and suicidal wishes and fantasies are consciously available to the pregnant woman (and to the professional, just for the asking . . .). However, they usually come wrapped in a reassurance: "Of course I wouldn't do anything now that I am pregnant." In this regard, it is of interest that at least one study mentions the frequency of suicidal threats and attempts in pregnant teen-agers, contrasted with the low incidence of "success" in this area (Gabrielson, Chapter 11).

BIOLOGICAL, PSYCHOLOGICAL, AND SOCIOCULTURAL TASKS OF PREGNANCY

The homeostasis of the woman is upset, physiologically, psychologically, and socially, as she moves through the transitional stage of pregnancy. It is still a moot question to what degree the emotional changes experienced by the pregnant and postpartum woman have a physiological basis, or to what extent they are a reflection of sociocultural or psychodynamic stresses.

Biological Considerations

> Pregnancy is a normal process, which, if it takes place under normal conditions of health and nutrition, is not harmful to the mother; certain interactions between her and the fetus become established which are even beneficial to her. In spite of this optimistic view having all too obvious social utility, however, gestation is a fatiguing task of no individual benefit to the woman, but on the contrary demanding heavy sacrifices . . . . All that a healthy and well-nourished woman can hope for is to recoup these losses without too much difficulty after childbirth [de Beauvoir, 1968].

The understanding of the physiological changes that make pregnant women a "species apart" have kept pace with the technology of modern medicine (Friedman, 1978). It is hoped a more intimate understanding of the changes in the milieu controlled by the hypothalamic, endocrine, and autonomic nervous systems will bring further light on the interplay of psychological and physiological changes in pregnancy. How much does the changed hormonal climate affect the woman's emotional state? Is there a physiological basis for the heightened awareness of "inner" life and for the sense of detachment from the outside world, the altered sense of self, the emotional lability, as well as for the passivity in terms of "acting" on the often strong ambivalent feelings that pregnant women experience during pregnancy? What is the role of the radical physiological changes as the woman is catapulted into the postpartum state, to again revert to "normal"? How do emotions interact with the neuroendocrine system? How are social stresses reflected in biochemical changes, and vice versa: how are chemical changes reflected in the way the self and the environment are perceived and related to? (Fuchs and Klopper, 1976; Donaldson, 1978; Daly, 1980).

The data on what, if any, relationship there is between the maternal psychological state and the behavior and function of the newborn child are fragmentary at best. We know that the fetus is exposed to the biochemical milieu of the mother, whether iatrogenically altered, or "naturally" through her own endocrine changes, establishing a neuroendocrine bond between them. In this context, it is of note that many of the psychoactive medications in use today, as well as other drugs misused or abused by the pregnant woman, are of concern in terms of their possible behavioral teratogenesis (Tylden, 1977; Donaldson, 1978; Lewis, 1978; Golub and Golub, 1981).

Sociocultural issues The social impact of a pregnancy as a major stressful life event has recently received more attention in the literature that has tended to emphasize either biological or psychodynamic issues (Shiness, 1966; Bibring and Valenstein, 1976; Turneer and Izzi, 1978; Oakley, 1980; Youngs and Lucas, 1980). Some of the obstacles or stress points in the journey from prepregnancy to motherhood can be conceptualized as:

1. Assuming the full adult role in our society, especially so with the first pregnancy. The woman will have to relinquish aspects of a dependent role and assume responsibility for the welfare of another.
2. A status passage, a point of no return, as the woman moves from the role of being an individual woman to that of becoming a mother. "From now on I have a new name, I'm no longer just Judy, but also 'Mom.' I have to practice it, it sounds so unfamiliar . . ." in the words of one of my patients.
3. Retirement may be one of the stresses, if a woman has been working, studying, or involved in building a career which she decides to cut down or off. This may well contribute to a sense of loss, change, and depression.
4. An occupational change, especially so with the first pregnancy, can involve considerable stress. In our society, many women will have their first contact with live babies when they hold their own. This often raises fears of not being able to cope or of hurting the baby through inexperience.

5. A change in the physical state, and the continuous adaptation required in this regard, presents the woman with its own particular stress.
6. Becoming a patient, often for the first time, the woman has to assume a new role as she turns to the medical profession, frequently with feelings of apprehension, helplessness, loss of control, and dependency. The increased technology (eg, frequent monitoring, sonograms, amniocentesis) over the past decades has greatly magnified the stresses of this aspect of pregnancy.
7. The approaching disaster event of labor and delivery is viewed during the pregnancy with increasing anxiety, and, afterwards, often leaves the woman with aftereffects similar to any other massive stress event. (This letdown may be related to the postpartum blues just as much as the rapidly changing hormones.)
8. The experience of hospitalization, being in an institution, separated from the family, and exposed to medical and surgical interventions.

Taken together, these stresses contribute to the heightened anxiety of pregnancy.

Another myth, which deserves to be laid to rest, is that the first pregnancy is the most stressful one. This, too, has been based on the finding that severe postpartum psychoses tend to be more common after a first pregnancy. But if we focus on slightly lesser degrees of psychological stress, it is evident that it is the multiparous mother who has the hardest time (Cohen, 1973; Hatherly et al, 1979; Oakley, 1980). Not only does she know from experience that pregnancy, childbirth, and early mothering are stressful, but she often gets less attention from the family, she has more daily responsibilities, and she is often overworked.

The women most vulnerable to perinatal morbidity, physical or psychological, tend to present with one or several social vulnerability factors: lack of confiding relationship with husband or boyfriend, having three or more children at home under the age of 14, having lost a mother before the age of 11, not being employed, having inadequate housing, having scant financial resources, and being socially isolated with an absence of a supportive network of family and friends (Wenner et al, 1969; Harvey, 1978; Oakley, 1980). An interesting aside, which may help explain some of the sense of differentness experienced by the pregnant woman, is a finding that pregnancy, in a sense, presents a "social stigma" in our society. Pregnant women tend to "become their role," and are treated differently from their prepregnant state. They are avoided, stared at, and not dealt with on as intimate a level as before (Taylor and Langer, 1977).

Psychodynamic Issues

The psychodynamic issues have been discussed by several authors with a psychoanalytic perspective (Heiman, 1965; Colman, 1969, 1971; Benedek, 1970; Bibring and Valenstein, 1976). I will review them in the context of the various stages of pregnancy, as the familiar conflicts of ambivalence towards the pregnancy, unresolved feelings towards one's mother, the struggle between emotional regression and progression, "regression in the service of the species," the increased dependency needs, and the issues related to pregnancy as a developmental phase in a woman's life, emerge.

The stage of motivation The period of decision making as to whether or not to become pregnant has become of increasing importance in our era of good contraceptive availability, abortion, and changing societal attitude towards bringing children into an already overpopulated world. Conflicts with familiar themes that will recur at later stages of pregnancy start surfacing, as the wish for a child struggles with the fears, hostilities, and negative feelings that work against it. The recurrent "leitmotif" is the woman's relationship with her mother. In exploring the motivation for pregnancy or the difficulties that stand in the way of successful pregnancy (infertility, miscarriages, ambivalences), there is often a regression to an earlier ambivalent mother–daughter relationship. There is the wish to have someone to love and be loved by, to be connected in a symbiotic way, to have a guaranteed love-object. Sometimes the pregnancy is seen as a gift to the partner, a wish to save a marriage, or a way to solidify or prove a sexual identity—repeating themes from the oedipal stage of development. In adolescents, pregnancy may express a wish to separate from the parents or to offer the baby as a present to the parents, eg, presenting the father with the boy he never had. Frequently it represents a wish to replace a lost love-object, a mother who recently died, a brother, a friend, a baby that was lost.

I am reminded of a woman who desperately wanted to get pregnant in the wake of her mother's and brother's death, struggling with a sense of a biological imperative in the face of realistic reasons not to become pregnant (age, work, husband's negative attitude). Unfortunately, unrealistic expectations of what needs or wishes the baby will fulfill can lead to negative emotional reactions, as the reality of pregnancy and infancy unfold. The most positive climate for a successful pregnancy occurs when a woman has good ego strength, when there is an absence of risk factors and a feeling that it "is the right time," when a woman has an understanding, loving husband and family, a good relationship with her mother, a supportive social network, and good financial resources. Today the issues around becoming pregnant stretch well into the first trimester, as the pregnant woman struggles with the decision to keep or not to keep the baby.

The first trimester The second stage has been termed "incorporating the reality of being pregnant" (Turneer and Izzi, 1978) and roughly coincides with the first trimester. An occasional woman never does master this stage, and delivers a baby whose existence has been denied by herself and others, up to the moment of active labor. In most women, there is a slow trickling in of information, such as missing a period, having a positive pregnancy test, seeing a physician. The early physiological changes of pregnancy—fatigue, nausea, gastrointestinal symptoms—often bring ambivalent feelings to the surface. It is during this stage that previous abortions or miscarriages can start haunting a woman. One woman, finally happily pregnant after months of trying, was shocked by her sudden fears that something terrible would happen to the baby, as well as by a frightening recurrent dream of being forcibly aborted—a mocking voice in the background stating: "You liked it before—why are you struggling now?"

Even under the most favorable circumstances, the actual impact of being pregnant tends to come as a shock. One woman tested her own urine one morning. When she saw the desired positive result, she surprised herself by feeling totally numb and going back to bed, unable to face the day. She felt that she had to "delay the reaction," there was so much to think about, to feel. "I have to deal with it first within myself, before I can deal with other people." This is not an unusual course of events: first the reality is incorporated within the self, then it is shared with the partner, later with the family, and even later, with friends. It took the woman in the above example a few days before she told her friends, and several weeks before she informed her colleagues at work about the happy event.

During this period the pregnant woman is often surprised by new fears and anxieties, perhaps an unusual interest in catastrophes and accidents, a sense of vulnerability and concern about getting hurt, or specific phobias, such as fear of driving, fears of open spaces, of bridges. Emotional lability is part of the picture, a sense of loss of emotional control, of crying more easily, of easily feeling embarrassed. Women tend to feel more in touch with their fantasies, more aware of and more involved with their bodies. They have a hovering kind of concern, coupled with a sense of loss of body boundaries, a loss of control over the body, which at times can be very frightening. As one woman put it, "I'm so afraid. . . . I'm afraid I'll lose control—that my body will be out of control." She increased her exercise program, and she started to diet, in an attempt to increase her sense of mastery in the face of "the inevitable fact that my body will take over. . . . It's like the whole fabric of my life has suddenly changed, the bearings are giving way. I have to change myself, my whole role. I'm also worried about being trapped in this mother-housewife role, maybe even liking it, sinking into it."

The second trimester As we move to the second trimester, the baby starts to become a reality. The preoccupation with the self—how pregnancy will affect one's body, one's life, one's future and relationships—gives way to an increasing awareness of the reality of the baby within. The relationship with the future child as a separate human being is the new focus, alongside the previous concerns. If a woman has not, until then, been consciously aware of feelings about her own mother, this is the phase during which they will emerge. There tends to be a reopening, a reawakening, of the mother–daughter relationship; she remembers, dreams about, talks about early feelings. If the mother is alive, she will often seek her out. If the mother is not available, or especially if she is dead, this can be a difficult time for the pregnant woman. A rejecting relationship with the mother can bring painful, ambivalent feelings to the fore.

New fears emerge during this period: fears for the baby, concerns about the content of the womb, about what is going on down there. This is the time for naming the baby. The mother who gives the baby an affectionate nickname (Pumpkin, Munchkin—or just plain "baby"), or a "real" name if she knows the sex of the child, is well on her way to include the new baby in her life. If the mother visualizes the fetus in negative terms, as a gnawing animal, a parasite, or as a cancerous growth, or if she has a sense of being taken over, raped from the inside, being controlled by this inner being, it bodes less well for the future. This is the stage of conscious symbiosis, of identification with self, with mother and baby all at the same time, inhabiting a private, special world.

Some comments from pregnant women: "I feel so good. I have more and more positive expectations. I'm aware on a subliminal level of the fact that the baby I miscarried a few months ago would have been born yesterday. I woke up this morning, half-asleep. When I touched my belly I was surprised that it was so small, I expected it to be nine-month's size. But I had a sense of relief. A baby would not fit into my schedule yet, it's too early. I was glad to have another five months to go." Another one: "I enjoy this feeling of slowing down. I used to be so afraid of stagnation. Now I look forward to being home, with a new awareness of how I've spent so much time denying to myself that I was a woman. I behaved 'as if I had a penis,' working and being so busy running around. Something about having a baby makes me feel different. I can't put it into words, but I have a new definition of myself as a woman." She described how she would check herself every day, feeling pleased and surprised by every change, occasionally shaking herself out of her contented state by saying: "This is all very nice, but remember, remember, there will be a real baby here."

Normative studies indicate that sexual activity and sexual interest decline steadily throughout pregnancy (Butler et al, 1979). The only dissenting voice is Masters' and Johnson's, who report an increase during the second trimester, perhaps explained by their volunteer population with a higher than usual interest in sexuality (Masters and Johnson, 1966). One woman expresses a "typical" reaction to sexuality in pregnancy:

> I feel I have an increased sexual awareness. I have all sorts of sexual fantasies, which is new to me. I have sexual dreams, sometimes with orgasm. The orgasms are often strong and powerful, but it's all sort of very distant. I feel as if my husband is a faceless stranger. When he says, 'let's make love!' I think of being pregnant, not sex, as if sex were in another world and another time. There is more awareness of my sexuality, of my body, but so much energy goes into this baby. She is in control, she's the center of the universe. Sometimes I feel so lonely, as if I am the only one in the world.

Many women experience a heightened awareness of sexuality and sensuality, and at the same time a withdrawing from close relationships into a universe alone with the baby.

Another woman expresses more concerns:

> There are so many fears on all sides, so many dilemmas. Should I go to work, should I continue my education? There is a sense of urgency, a need to sort it all out. I am afraid of doing something harmful, harming my child, my marriage, myself. I'm so afraid of being abandoned, because I've become so dependent. Pregnancy changes you, everyone sees you differently. My mother-in-law sees me as the bearer of her grandchild, my friends as a mother. No other crisis, such as leaving for school, marrying, moving, has felt like this. This is so monumentally different. I have never felt so changed. Once in a while I can feel very happy, as if I am in the mainstream with the baby—or caught in a mystery, while the rest of the world goes on outside us.

Another woman had an ongoing inner dialogue with her mother, who was dead. "Sometimes I sit and rattle with her for hours, just wishing to be close, to share. . . . In the next moment I will feel furious with her, and find myself yelling out loud: 'I ain't gonna be like you mother!' Then I laugh, because she was such a stickler for grammar . . ."

The last trimester The last trimester presents yet another theme, the impending separation, as labor looms increasingly at the horizon. Fears tend to come back in full force. New decisions, new conflicts, new fears emerge as the woman senses the end of the journey, the "crash down" in sight. Worries about delivery, anesthesia, helplessness in the face of the inevitable event come to the forefront. Women often become preoccupied with death, they watch accidents on television, they find themselves morbidly interested in news stories about disasters. "I feel so vulnerable, it's a strange new feeling. I've lost control of the central core of myself." Working as a social worker, she finds it hard to work with adolescents and their mothers:

> I'm so diffuse nowadays. I don't know whom I identify with. Is it the mother, the daughter? Sometimes I decide that I identify with both, I feel like both mother and daughter at the same time. . . . I also find that I've suddenly become more aware of separation issues. I guess separation is a big issue for me right now. . . . I have so many things to worry about . . . separating from the baby, separating from my former self, separating from being pregnant, separating from work. It's too much!

And another woman: "For months I used to talk about delivery, and I maintained that I wasn't the least bit worried. Ha!! The bigger I get, the closer to due date I get, the more I think about how hard delivery will be. I even had the fear the other day that I was going to die on the delivery table. When I talked with my husband about it, I wish I hadn't. He got so freaked out and clingy, I couldn't stand it."

The fear of death sometimes continues right into delivery, causing some terrifying emotional experiences. One woman recalled her first pregnancy as a teen-ager, how petrified she was during delivery. She was convinced that she was going to die . . . she was too frightened to scream. When they put her to sleep, she thought, "Well, this is how they are going to get me. My parents want to get rid of me and the doctors are doing it for them." Another woman had a recurrent dream, where she was rolled into the delivery room, the delivery table draped in black, an ominous voice saying: "You're next!"

The postpartum period The postpartum period is one of a labile, depressed mood, as the postpartum "blues" affect the majority of women, at least briefly during the two to five days after delivery. One woman with a very mild reaction states one week postpartum: "It feels as if I'm in a dream. Sometimes I feel great, the next moment it can be really bad and horrifying. But every day I feel that I can relax more and more." After another week, she adds: "It was so natural and easy, I would do it again."

Others feel more of an ego-depletion, a loss, an incapacity to tolerate one more thing, feeling stretched to their capacity. A woman experiencing a couple of weeks of "let-down": "I miss that sensuous awareness of my baby. I am much less aware now. I remind myself, I should be happy, I'm not pregnant, it's all over. I lost some muscles, I have put on some extra weight. I had a pretty good delivery, but I was annoyed at the epidural and the forceps. I was relieved that I had an orgasm during sex. I must have been unconsciously afraid, worried that my body had changed. I feel that I am older. It's so difficult to divide your love between so many people."

Still another woman with a hidden postpartum reaction that she only talked about a year later:

> I was petrified all the time, walking about in a dreamlike state. I was fearful that the baby wasn't breathing, wasn't eating right, wasn't gaining weight. Worried that there was something wrong with the food, that it was too old, too cold, would cause botulism. Afraid to look out the window, for fear I would throw out the baby. Afraid to go out in the street, for fear I would push the carriage in front of a car by accident—afraid, afraid—and most of all afraid of saying anything to anyone, because I felt so guilty and ashamed of my terrible thoughts.

DISCUSSION

The mystery remains. Pregnant women are more intensely aware of their emotions, experiencing a wide range of affects, fluctuating from moments of despair to periods of peaceful or excited coexistence with the world. They experience high levels of anxiety, mood disorders, and psychological stress states throughout their pregnancies, yet severe psychiatric manifestations are rare, including suicide. Are these intensified negative feelings offset by an equally expanded range of positive, joyful feelings?

Are the explanations to be found in deeper understanding of the neuroendocrine changes during pregnancy—do they have a naturally tranquilizing effect on the mother?

Does the sociocultural role of a pregnant woman offer some protection from these inner anxieties and conflicts? Does the pregnant woman suppress the expression of anxieties as she conforms to the role expected of her in our culture? Does the fact that pregnancy covers a finite time span, that there is an end in sight, delay or inhibit acting out impulses? Does the woman respond to a deeper calling, feeling that she has to preserve herself in the service of the species?

Is the awareness that suicide during pregnancy also involves homicide a deterrent to expressing self-destructive impulses?

Does the physical and psychological symbiosis with the fetus inhibit any impulses of destruction—the mother identifying with the fetus, as well as with herself and with her own mother?

The questions and quest for answers remain.

CHAPTER 13

POSTPARTUM MENTAL ILLNESS

BONNIE SAKS

INTRODUCTION/EPIDEMIOLOGY

As Dr. Kleiner and others have found, suicide during pregnancy is extremely rare. Psychiatric illness during the first three months postpartum, however, is extraordinarily common. The added risk for admission to mental hospitals for psychosis is 3.0 to 3.6 per 1000 women (Pugh et al, 1963), or three to five times normal. The incidence of depression in women, in general, is well documented to be twice that of men (Weissman and Klerman, 1977; Guttentag et al, 1980; Carmen et al, 1981). The incidence of depression in women postpartum increases five- to sevenfold, and is 10–20% in most studies (Pitt, 1968; Braverman and Roux, 1978; Paykel et al, 1980). Of those women who are depressed and untreated, Pitt (1968) found that 40–50% remain persistently depressed after one year.

A more mild, transient depression called "postpartum blues," occurs in 60–80% of all women postpartum (Pitt, 1968; Yalom et al, 1968; Braverman and Roux, 1978).

Although very few of the women who become psychotic or severely depressed actually commit suicide (in fact, depressed patients without psychotic features most often are not admitted to hospitals), the mental illness can be disabling to the mother, to her relationships, and significantly, to the development of her children (Bibring and Valenstein, 1976).

Certainly, postpartum mental illness is a highly prevalent problem. Why then is it not given more attention?

When a woman has a psychotic illness postpartum, her behavior is usually too flagrant to be ignored and she is hospitalized. Indeed women are hospitalized for psychotic illness at a five times higher rate postpartum than at any other time in the life cycle (Pugh et al, 1963). Hospitalization of men does not show this increased incidence after a baby is born, although anecdotal cases of men hospitalized after a birth are reported.

The most striking findings in terms of incidence are the extremely high percentages of women with postpartum blues, 60% by Saks et al (to be published) at Yale of women with no previously known psychiatric or medical illness, and 60% also by Yalom et al (1968) at Stanford and by Braverman and Roux (1978) in Montreal.

The numbers are impressive but, although the phenomena may cause discomfort, it is transient and people recover without treatment. If there are any lasting ill effects, these are not determined.

The high incidence of clinical depression, 10% or greater, as found by Braverman and Roux (1978), Pitt (1968) and Saks et al (to be published) is of great concern. These depressed women usually do not have suicidal attempts or call attention loudly enough to their dysfunction to become hospitalized or ensure treatment. Half of them are still not functioning well after a year, and the sequela on the family occur insidiously. Sometimes the illness is brought to attention by another family member's distress, eg, the baby may present with failure to thrive because the mother is giving sometimes inadequate physical, and more often, inadequate emotional nourishment. More often, a marginal functioning persists where life goes on, but healthy personal and interpersonal growth may be impaired.

DEFINITION OF TERMS

In order to understand and study the different courses, possible etiologies, and most efficacious treatment of postpartum mental illness, the different types of syndromes must be consistently defined.

The obstetric literature is particularly confusing, often lumping widely disparate syndromes into one poorly defined category.

Only recently (1980) has the American Psychiatric Association published the third edition of the *Diagnostic and Statistical Manual of Mental Disorders* (DSM-III), the standard reference for defining syndromes by clinical criteria.

Psychosis

Postpartum psychotic reactions include the following spectrum of illnesses: schizophrenoform disorder, brief reactive psychosis, atypical psychosis, major affective disorder, and organic brain syndrome.

The psychotic features which any of these may have are: (1) behavior that is grossly disorganized or catatonic, (2) bizarre delusions such as being controlled, controlling others, (3) religious or somatic hallucinations, and (4) incoherence or loosening of associations.

A schizophrenoform reaction has at least one of the above and has lasted more than two weeks. A brief reactive psychosis lasts less than two weeks and is an immediate reaction to a stressful event. An atypical psychosis is the category most postpartum psychoses fall into, since they often do not meet the criteria for other forms of psychosis. When the person has no previous history of psychotic symptoms but develops a very unusual presentation such as a single delusion about bodily change or persistent auditory hallucinations without other functional impairment, the diagnosis is atypical psychosis. This type of psychosis may indeed be subtle enough to be overlooked by a casual observer, especially when the woman appears psychotic only when questioned about her one symptom.

A postpartum manic-depressive psychosis, on the other hand, rarely goes unnoticed. Studies have indicated that people with manic-depressive illness [mood swings of "highs" with racing thoughts, hyperactivity, and grandiosity, to lows of clinical depression (to be defined later)] have a special risk for an episode to occur in the puerperium. Also, having had an affective postpartum episode makes a future postpartum episode more likely (Reich and Winokur, 1970; Wintour et al, 1980).

A study at the University of Iowa suggested that women with postpartum mania have fewer recurrent episodes outside the postpartum period and more Schneiderian (psychotic) symptoms (Kadrmas et al, 1979). One example cited is a 26-year-old woman who "felt that her home doctor had hypnotized her and had a power over her so that he could impose strange things on her. For instance, he made her skin itchy and made her want him."

There is much debate about drug treatment for manic-depressive, psychotic, and depressed patients prenatally and postpartum, especially with lithium, an invaluable drug for treatment of mania but with known teratogenic effects for the fetus and other ill effects when transmitted through breast milk (Schoum and Amdisen, 1973).

Case report Patient K was 37 years old and married two years prior to this first pregnancy. She was hospitalized for acute mania at age 14 and was rehospitalized numerous times for manic episodes until age 28, when she was admitted to the NIMH inpatient research program. Her history also included severe depressive episodes without hospitalization. She was discharged from an NIMH inpatient unit on lithium carbonate and followed for medication supervision and weekly psychotherapy in an NIMH outpatient clinic. In the seven post-hospital discharge years, the patient experienced mild mood changes without impairment, and a brief appearance of manic symptoms only during participation in an off-lithium research protocol. Otherwise, patient K had been essentially euthymic for seven years while taking lithium. She voluntarily discontinued lithium five weeks before she became pregnant. At the time of the birth, patient K had been off lithium for 10 months.

Patient K worked until her last month, when she became fatigued, and showed no overt symptoms of affective illness throughout the pregnancy. In the last week, patient K expressed impatience and restlessness.

> Patient K delivered a boy via caesarean section after a difficult labor and reported that the experience had been very trying for her. She chose to breast-feed and returned home with the infant at one week. On the 10th postpartum day, patient K called to inform us that she felt that she was becoming hypomanic, and requested reinstitution of lithium carbonate in order to avert hospitalization. Upon examination, the patient appeared overtalkative, restless and somewhat hyperactive, easily distractable, increasingly grandiose, more dramatic and assertive, and moderately euphoric. She described a decreased need for sleep and a desire to make many telephone calls. She was treated immediately with thioridazine for one week and restarted on lithium carbonate. With the support of her husband and therapist, patient K ceased breast-feeding, maintained minimal child-care responsibility, and was euthymic within one week [Targum et al, 1979].

As will be discussed later in the section on etiology, it is not clear in this case what importance the external support system had compared to the lithium. There is a good discussion of proper treatment and medication use in obstetric and gynecologic patients with affective illness in the article "What can you do for the depressed patient?" (Saks, 1981).

Blues

Postpartum blues is a very prevalent condition but also one which is defined differently by different people. Since "blues" is a transient condition that does not usually necessitate treatment, it is important to distinguish it from the more serious postpartum illnesses such as depression, which should be recognized and treated.

Most researchers have defined the postpartum blues syndrome to be a very mild form of depression characterized by prolonged crying, irritability, fatigue, and occurring within the first two weeks postpartum (Treadway et al, 1969; Paykel et al, 1980). Yet, the period of "blues" does not commence before two or three days postpartum, usually sometime after the patient has returned home (Braverman and Roux, 1978; Paykel et al, 1980). According to this definition, independent investigators (Yalom at Stanford, Pitt in London, Braverman and Roux in Montreal, and Saks and Frank at Yale) have found the incidence to be around 60%.

Anecdotally, Saks and her coworkers at Yale and many obstetricians noted a phenomenon earlier than the "blues syndrome," a period of very labile emotion, tearfulness not associated with sad or depressed moods. Most women seen within the first two days postpartum commented on this phenomenon, eg, "I just start crying watching TV or walking around, but I'm not sad." This experience should not be confused with "blues."

Depression

A much more serious illness, also not beginning until sometime after the woman has returned home from the hospital, is postpartum depression.

There is no precise diagnostic category in DSM-III, but Saks et al (to be published) have defined postpartum depression as meeting the criteria for a major depressive episode, which are:

A. Dysphoric mood: at least two weeks duration
B. At least four of the following:
   1. Poor appetite or weight loss or significant weight gain
   2. Insomnia or hypersomnia
   3. Psychomotor agitation or retardation
   4. Loss of interest or pleasure in usual activities
   5. Loss of energy
   6. Feelings of worthlessness, self-reproach or excessive guilt
   7. Diminished ability to think or concentrate
   8. Suicidal thoughts

Instruments based on the criteria measuring depression in the general population, such as the self-rating Beck Depression Inventory, have been tested in large population studies and also seem to validly measure depression in postpartum patients according to current work by Saks et al (to be published). With the physiologic symptoms of weight loss and sleep interruption (eg, to feed the baby), not all measures of depression are accurate in the puerperium, and because some depressive symptoms are dismissed as physiologic (eg, fatigue, loss of appetite, insomnia), an accurate diagnosis is often missed. The true incidence of puerperal depression, as mentioned, is about 10% of women (Pitt, 1968), and these women are at some risk for suicide. The children of these mothers may also be at risk.

ETIOLOGIES

Certainly, the postpartum mental disorders are a heterogeneous group and may have widely different or mixed etiologies.

Endocrine

Many heated debates have gone on about "the great hormonal changes" in women and whether or not they affect their psyches. Let us examine the specific hormones during pregnancy and the puerperium and think about what psychological affects might result postpartum.

Human chorionic gonadotropin (HCG) is a glycoprotein produced by the syncytiotrophoblast. It shares the same subunit as luteinizing hormone (LH), follical stimulating hormone (FSH), and thyroid stimulating hormone (TSH). The half-life ($t\,½$) is 24 hours.

Urine HCG is the current index for determination of pregnancy. Now, the more accurate (less cross-reacting material) beta-subunit blood test can determine pregnancy nine days after conception. The beta-HCG radioimmunoassay eliminates the spuriously high values for HCG by other methods.

HCG peaks at 60–70 days gestation (Pritchard and MacDonald, 1976). Higher titers are reached with multiple fetuses, and highest titers with hydatidiform moles, but there is no dramatic change later in pregnancy (Braunstein et al, 1976). If HCG affected mood or thought processes, it most likely would have its most potent effect around 60 days or so gestation, not postpartum.

Human placental lactogen (HPL), a single polypeptide chain, is detectable in the trophoblast by the third week postovulation. Like HCG, it is concentrated in the syncytiotrophoblast (which becomes the placenta) and rises during the first and second trimesters proportional to placental mass. By the third trimester, it reaches levels higher than any other protein hormone. $t\,½ = 25$ minutes.

HPL reaches levels of 6000 ng/mL at term, 30 times prolactin levels. Postpartum HPL levels decline in a biphasic manner, initially $t½ =$ 12–14.5 minutes, and a second more prolonged $t½ = 40$ minutes.

Estrogens As early as the seventh week gestation, more than 50% of the estrogens entering the maternal circulation are produced by the placenta, and the placenta continues to be the major site of estrogen production in pregnancy.

Estriol, the estrogen produced by the placenta, accounts for almost all of the total stable estrogen measurable during the latter weeks of pregnancy.

High estriol excretion is seen in multiple pregnancies, Rh-positive mother with Rh-negative fetus, and theoretically, with fetal adrenal hyperplasia prior to delivery (the last five weeks). Concordant with prolactin increase and fetal adrenal growth, estrogen production increases greatly. Following delivery, when the placental production site is removed, there is a precipitous fall in estrogens (Hay, 1976).

A number of studies have indicated that estrogen may enhance central adrenergic functioning.

1. Administration of ethinyl estradiol to female mice pretreated with monoamine oxidase inhibitors (MAOIs) resulted in increased norepinephrine (NE) content in various portions of the brain (Klaiber et al, 1979). Might estrogen then increase norepinephrine synthesis?

2. Catechol estrogens, metabolites of estradiol (E_2) have been reported to competitively inhibit enzymatic methylation and biological inactivation of NE by catecho-*o*-methyl transferase (COMT) (Klaiber et al, 1979); E_2 might potentiate NE action.

3. Estrogens inhibit monoamine oxidase activity both in rat hypothalamus and human plasma (Klaiber et al, 1979). Might then estrogen make NE more available?

Assuming that the catecholamine deficiency hypothesis for explaining depression is correct, estrogen theoretically could have an antidepressant action and lowered estrogen might increase depression.

Progesterone Like estrogen, the placenta becomes the major site of progesterone production (after the tenth week). The major metabolite is pregnanediol. For progesterone production, fetal contribution is minimal.

Near parturition, there is a decline in progesterone concentration coincident with increased resting potential (myometrial contractability) of the uterus. Thus by about 34 weeks, progesterone begins a rapid decline. The course of decline does not correlate in time with the onset of depressed mood.

Human chorionic adrenocorticotropic hormone (ACTH) There is much evidence for placental ACTH which may account for free cortisol rise in the placenta during pregnancy and may stimulate both maternal adrenal activity and fetal adrenal hyperplasia, but the rise is not dramatic nor is the postpartum decline.

Prolactin is increased in pregnancy up to 2000 ng/mL at term. The initial rise at seven to eight weeks correlates with increased estradiol (which acts at the hypothalamus to increase prolactin). Prolactin does not pass through the placenta. Measurement of prolactin is the same in variability as in the nonpregnant state, peaking four to five hours after sleep.

Prolactin is most interesting. Despite its short $t\frac{1}{2}$, prolactin levels decline over seven days postpartum in the non-breast-feeding mother. Suckling causes transient prolactin inhibitory hormone (PIF) inhibition, thus increased prolactin (PIF may be dopamine).

There are anecdotal reports of depression accompanying weaning, and the course of prolactin decline is in closer temporal relationship with the onset of depression, blues, and psychosis.

Growth hormone and the pituitary Growth hormone is low in pregnancy and remains low after delivery (Treadway et al, 1969).

The pituitary itself enlarges during pregnancy, although it is not an essential gland. Pregnancy has been maintained posthypophysectomy with corticosteroids, and thyroid, and vasopressin replacement.

Thyroid stimulating hormone (TSH) is unchanged during pregnancy as is unbound thyroxin (T_4). Because of increased estrogens, there is an increase in thyroxin binding proteins resulting in an elevated T_4 index and decreased triiodothyronine (T_3) uptake. The thyroid gland itself is enlarged in pregnancy because of increased vascularity.

It is interesting to keep in mind that thyroid releasing hormone (TRH) (from the hypothalamus) is a potent releasing factor for prolactin in opposition to dopamine. TRH is probably not changed in pregnancy.

Adrenocorticotropic hormone (ACTH) concentrations are decreased in the plasma of pregnant women, although these levels increase gradually as pregnancy progresses (Saks et al, to be published).

Cortisol, deoxycorticosterone (DOC), and aldosterone levels are increased in pregnancy. Aldosterone readily responds to salt balance and postural stimuli, and thus increases only to the extent of maintaining normal volume homeostasis. Cortisol rise, like T_4, may be secondary to increased binding proteins secondary to increased estrogens. ACTH does not cross the placenta. The existence of placental ACTH is still an open question.

There are very few studies which have actually measured endocrine values simultaneously with valid measurement of mood change or development of psychotic symptoms.

Nott et al (1976) did clinical interviews for data on personality and measured plasma levels of LH, FSH, total estrogen, progesterone, and prolactin in 27 normal pregnant women three times before delivery and 16 times during the six weeks following delivery. An attempt was made to correlate hormone findings and clinical findings. This attempt failed to produce any strong evidence that hormones are related to mood.

Similarly, Saks et al (to be published) administered standard self-rating scales to assess mood at 26 weeks and at 36 weeks gestation, and two days and six weeks postpartum. Simultaneously, blood samples were drawn for estradiol, progesterone, and prolactin; 24-hour urine was also collected for estriol. Subjects were 20 women with no history of significant psychiatric or medical illness. Again, there was no strong correlation that these hormone levels were related to depression or blues postpartum.

The sample sizes were small in both studies and the subjects were "normal" women, ie, no known psychiatric history. It may well be that women who are biochemically prone to depression or psychosis may show more response to hormonal flux. Only careful further research can determine this.

External Supports

Social supports Another area of etiologic research for postpartum mental illness is that of social support. Gordon and Gordon (1959), Wenner et al (1969), and others believe that pregnancy is a time when the degree of emotional support, particularly by the husband, is important.

In 1959, Gordon and Gordon did a study of 98 women postpartum whose physicians rated the degree of emotional disturbance. Thirty percent of the women experienced some degree of emotional upset. Responses of the women to a social history questionnaire given during the postpartum hospital stay were analyzed to evaluate differences in the social history of women who experienced no, slight, or much emotional upset during the subsequent postpartum period. Women who experienced postpartum emotional difficulties differed from women who did not with respect to factors in the wife's social history, the husband's social history, their marriage, physical complications of pregnancy, complications with children, and the absence of available help. Comparisons of responses from 55 psychiatric patients indicated that they also experienced the stressful social history events.

Having identified social factors associated with postpartum emotional problems, Gordon and Gordon (1960) designed this study to explore the value of adding preparation for parenthood information to the content of prenatal baby care classes and explored the effect of involvement of the expectant father in the classes. Class groups were randomly assigned to an experimental condition, receiving supplementary preparation for parenthood material described as follows:

1. The responsibilities of being a mother (and not a martyr) are learned, hence get help and advice.
2. Make friends of other couples who are experienced with young children.
3. Don't overload yourself with extra, less important tasks.
4. Don't move soon after the baby arrives.
5. Don't be too concerned with appearances when other things are more important.
6. Get plenty of rest and sleep.
7. Don't be a nurse to elderly relatives at this period.
8. Confer and consult with husband, family, and experienced friends and discuss your plans and worries.
9. Don't give up your outside interests, but cut down the responsibilities and rearrange your schedules.
10. Arrange for babysitters in advance.
11. Learn to drive a car.

Postpartum emotional problems were reduced by the preparation and by the participation of husbands: 11% of the women whose husbands attended classes and 23% of the women attending alone experienced postpartum emotional problems compared with 37% of the women in the control group. Six months later effects of the supplementary preparation persisted. Half the women were included in the six-month follow-up, at which time 2% of the experimental and 28% of the control group women were having problems.

Gordon and Gordon (1960) found that there were six areas of behavior change which were associated with a reduction in postpartum emotional problems:

1. They made more friends of couples with young children.
2. They gave less emphasis to tidiness in the home.
3. They obtained more experienced help with the baby.
4. The husband became more available in the home and reduced his outside activities.
5. The couple continued to socialize outside the home, but less frequently.
6. The wife continued with her outside interests, but limited her responsibilities.

Life stress Other investigators put more emphasis on stressful life events. Paykel et al (1980) found, of 120 women, there was a 20% prevalence of mild clinical depression at six weeks postpartum. This research indicated the strongest associated factor to be the occurrence of recent stressful life events. Poor marital support acted as a vulnerability factor, only producing an effect in the presence of stressful life events. Incidently, previous psychiatric history produced a strong independent effect both with and without life events (Paykel et al, 1980). Previous psychiatric history for depression or psychosis is a known risk factor both for postpartum depression and psychosis, respectively (Cohler et al, 1974).

Mother–baby interaction Another variable which should be considered apart from the mother's internal conflicts and hormonal status is the mother–baby match. Some mothers are more comfortable (or unhappy) with an intrinsically quiet baby, while others feel more stimulated (or more overwhelmed) with an active one. The effect of the infant's behavior on the mother and the mother's on the infant is very significant (Bardon, 1973).

Other physical factors Other nonhormonal possible physical determinants of mood include fatigue, lack of REM (rapid eye movement) sleep, and physical discomfort (overweight, episiotomy or cesarean section wound healing, engorged breasts, or cramps). It has been shown that there is decreased REM and stage 4 sleep in the first two months postpartum. It is also known that decreased REM sleep can eventually precipitate depression or psychosis in some cases. There are no specific studies, however, measuring stage 4 or REM sleep concurrently with mental state postpartum.

Internal Conflicts

Many authors have written about internal conflicts, particularly concerning the woman's relationship to her own mother, as being critical to her emotional adjustment postpartum.

Helene Deutch (1944–1945) described pregnancy as a state of crisis. Grete Bibring further considered that pregnancy is indeed a developmental crisis for all women (Bibring and Valenstein, 1976).

As others agree, pregnancy is a time of psychological disequilibrium. At such a time, there is maturational potential for new and adaptive solutions (Leifer, 1977).

Bibring observed that pregnant women were most preoccupied with their relationship with their own mother. The women in Bibring's study made spontaneous statements which referred to a change they sensed in their reaction to their mothers. She says, "It is as if the attitudes in this relationship established as solutions of childhood experiences are abandoned and replaced by various new forms of identification with the mother." In successful maturation, she says, the women develop a useful identity with the mother as the prototype parental figure (Bibring and Valenstein, 1976). When there is conflict about identifying with the mother, however, this useful identification may not occur. Some women can appreciate that they can become a different mother from their own, but one's own mother usually remains a predominant model. It is also hard for a mother to know how to invest in and bond with a baby if she hasn't been invested in and bonded with during her development.

In summary, factors which may contribute to depression, psychosis, and suicide potential are: lack of external support from husband, mother, and/or significant others, recent stressful life events, incompatible personality match between mother and baby, lack of early contact with baby (decreasing maternal attachment and investment), decreased REM and stage 4 sleep, physical discomfort or pain, and internal conflicts about assuming the role of "mother." There is some evidence that hormonal flux does not contribute to psychosis or depression in "normal" women. However, previous history of depression, psychosis, or suicidal gesturing predisposes to recurrence in the postpartum, and this group of women may be influenced by biochemical or hormonal changes.

PREDICTION/WOMEN AT RISK

As mentioned, it is already known that women with a previous history of mental illness may be at risk postpartum. We know, however, that the risk for serious depression postpartum is 10% in normal women. How can this group be predicted? Consideration of external stressors, supports, and internal conflicts about mothering are important. Based on some of these etiologic factors, Braverman and Roux (1978) designed a short 19-item questionnaire. Saks et al (to be published) gave this questionnaire to a small sample of normal women at 26 and 36 weeks gestation and found it highly predictive for depression by six weeks postpartum. There needs to be more testing on a larger scale. Hayworth et al (1980) noted that high anxiety and high hostility were associated with postpartum depression. Saks et al (to be published) noted in particular that anger directed inward was much greater for women who became depressed. Others have indicated that individuals with high hostility levels represent difficulties in handling interpersonal relationships, and anxiety (and depression) resulted from anticipated difficulty in handling the new baby (Brown and Harris, 1978). Others have indicated that such individuals have poor relationships with their husbands or mothers (Hayworth et al, 1980). There are studies in progress to determine if there are simpler ways for determining women at risk (Frommer and O'Shea, 1973; Braverman and Roux, 1978; Saks et al, to be published).

NEUROCHEMICAL MARKERS

It certainly would be advantageous if a simple biochemical analysis could be done to determine which women were ill and at risk at their six week check-up postpartum, especially for those depressed women who are not diagnosed and could benefit from treatment.

There has been a lot of interest in finding biochemical markers of psychiatric illness. The monoamine hypothesis of affective disorders articulated by Schildkrant and Kety (1965), states that "some, if not all, depressions may be associated with a relative deficiency of norepinephrine at receptor sites in the brain, while elation may be associated with an excess of this amine."

Evidence for this theory came from the observation that drugs which deplete norepinephrine centrally (eg, reserpine, alphamethyldopa) produce depression in 10–15% of people, especially if there is a history of previous depression (Maas, 1978). Drugs which antagonize reserpine can be effective antidepressant agents. Also, drugs which displace norepinephrine from binding sites in the brain, interfere with storage and uptake, or act as false transmitters have been associated with unusual mental phenomena, including psychosis (Jarrahi-Zadeh et al, 1969).

The main central nervous system metabolite of norepinephrine is 3-methoxy-4-hydroxyphenethylene glycol (MHPG), which is excreted in the urine (Sweeney and Maas, 1978). In studies measuring three-day urinary MHPG levels in bipolar depressed, depressed, and control subjects, bipolar depressed and depressed patients have lower MHPG than normals (Maas, 1978). The finding has important treatment implications which have been tested (Sweeney and Maas, 1978). Low MHPG levels are also found in some schizophrenic patients; this is not yet a reliable predictor of psychiatric diagnosis (Sweeney and Maas, 1978).

Saks et al (to be published) are currently measuring 24-hour urinary MHPG in pregnant and postpartum women. Other studies are finding out more about tryptophan, serotonin, and the relation of catecholestrogens to mood states. Perhaps there will soon be neurochemical markers to alert us to the postpartum woman at risk for depression, psychosis, suicide. Right now the best signs are clinical.

SUMMARY

The epidemiology of postpartum mental illness has been discussed, and the various syndromes defined. Postpartum blues is seen to be quite prevalent (upwards of 60%) but self-limited and not associated with suicide. Postpartum psychoses (about 0.2%) are a heterogeneous group of disorders and can be associated with suicide potential. Postpartum depression, although more rarely associated with suicide, is highly prevalent (10%) and has a high degree of morbidity if untreated.

The possible etiologies of postpartum mental disorders were discussed. In women without previous psychiatric history, there is no evidence of hormonal determinants. Whether there are certain women more susceptible to biochemical determinants is not yet known. Of the external variables that may be important, social support systems, especially a husband's support, life stresses, physical stresses, and maternal–child interaction seem to be significant. The woman's internal conflicts that permit or prevent her from accepting her baby and her new role as a mother, as well as her personality and ego functioning, may also be critical for development of postpartum dysfunction or maturation (Hayworth et al, 1980).

Current efforts and methods for prediction of women at risk as well as biochemical markers were discussed. Some research looks promising, but all tools should be used with caution.

Certainly, as Bibring and Valenstein (1976) said:

> Psychologically, childbirth remains for many young women a highly stressful experience, giving rise to deeply seated archaic anxieties beyond the reach of the advanced scope of today's medical techniques.
>
> Modern obstetrics would do well to become aware of this discrepancy. Instead of focusing exclusively on the physiologic management, it is essential that a good obstetric setting include full awareness and attention to the prevalent psychological attitudes, fears, and expectations of the pregnant woman. Optimally, she should feel that her obstetrician recognizes her as a person with her own individuality and outlook toward pregnancy and motherhood.

CHAPTER 14

POSTPARTUM PSYCHIATRIC SYNDROMES

NICHOLAS DESTOUNIS

Postpartum mental illness was first clinically described by Hippocrates in the 4th century BC. In the Third Book of the Epidemics, he cited the case of a woman who gave birth to twins, experienced severe insomnia and restlessness on the sixth day postpartum, became delirious on the eleventh day, then comatose, and died on the seventeenth day.

In 1838, Esquirol dispelled a great deal of the mysticism surrounding the disease, and during the remainder of the 19th century considerable interest in the problem arose.

Marce's (1858) outstanding book, *Traité de la folie des femmes enceintes; des nouvelles accouchées et des nourrices*, is perhaps the only comprehensive book in the world literature on the subject.

In 1942, Boyd emphasized the importance of the psychological, physical, physiological, and social stresses imposed upon the pregnant woman.

Brew (1950), in his studies on postpartum psychoses, found that 14% had a family history of psychosis, and in 60% a definite personality makeup could be determined; 23% of the patients gave a history of a mental disorder associated with a previous parturition.

Hamilton (1962) tends to favor the physiological etiology of these syndromes.

The central thesis of this communication is that psychosociophysiological factors play an important role in the development of the postpartum psychiatric syndromes.

CLINICAL PICTURE—ETIOLOGY

The clinical picture of a postpartum psychiatric syndrome varies greatly, and it is rather difficult to diagnose with certainty whether a patient presents symptoms of an acute schizophrenic reaction, manic-depressive reaction, or borderline psychosis (severe obsessive neurosis with phobias).

Several investigators have reported that the presence of delirium in postpartum psychiatric illness varies from 28 to 34%. If we are to accept that the symptom delirium accompanies its clinical picture, then we ought to examine the whole of this subject from a pathophysiological viewpoint, for in most cases the symptoms of confusion and delirium are signs of an organic syndrome (metabolic, toxic, chemical, nutritional, etc). At this particular point a very important question arises: Do the postpartum psychiatric syndromes develop only due to a disturbance of the physiological equilibrium of the organism? This cannot be accepted for the following reasons:

1. We believe that the etiology of the postpartum mental illness is a psychosociophysiological one.
2. Our experience has shown us that the symptoms of confusion and delirium do not always accompany its clinical picture.
3. We believe that, as the minor or major pregnancy complications can be prevented by psychotherapeutic means, the same can be achieved with this syndrome, providing the chymes of the organism are normal (Destounis, 1962, 1964a,b).

OBJECTIVES

A. To determine the physiological, psychological, and socioeconomic factors associated with the postpartum mental illness.
B. To establish the incidence of an organic pathology (confusion, delirium) in postpartum psychiatric syndromes.
C. The relationship between A and B.

HYPOTHESES

1. That psychosociophysiological factors are associated with the postpartum psychiatric syndromes.
2. That the organic symptomatology (confusion, delirium) does not necessarily accompany a postpartum psychiatric illness.
3. That the incidence of a schizophrenic-like postpartum illness is higher than any other postpartum mental illness.

METHODOLOGY

To accomplish the objectives of our study, arrangements were made so that all the admitted patients with a history of a postpartum mental illness were seen, interviewed, and treated by the author. A complete medical-obstetrical and psychiatric history was obtained which included father's and husband's socioeconomic status, dwelling data, religion, age, education, nationality, etc. Furthermore, the physical examination and investigation included a complete laboratory work-up including protein-bound iodine (PBI).

STUDY GROUP

We are presenting here the study group of 26 patients who were seen in different psychiatric wards of general and state hospitals between the years 1955 and 1963 in the United States and Canada.

RESULTS AND ANALYSIS

The findings of this group are presented in Table 14-1 which illustrates the psychiatric diagnosis and social classification of the total group of 26 women. Thus, 15 of the patients were classified as paranoid schizophrenics whose clinical picture was as follows: paranoid ideas with delusions, auditory hallucinations, depression, dissociations, unrealistic thinking, inappropriate affect, etc. Five were classified as manic-depressives whose clinical picture was as follows: elation with flight of ideas, unlimited confidence (manic phase), or motor retardation, guilt feelings, depression, self-accusations, loss of self-esteem, obsessional thinking, self-depreciation, suicidal ideas, insomnia (depressed phase). Five were classified as nonpsychotics, but clinically they presented symptoms of a mild depression accompanied by obsessional thinking and phobias. One was classified as schizophrenic (schizoaffective type) with profound impairment of both ego and superego.

Table 14-1
Clinical Diagnosis and Subjects Class Identification

Diagnosis	Social Classification*		Number
Schizophrenic reaction (paranoid type)	I and II	5	15
	III	5	
	IV and V	5	
Manic-depressive reaction (depressed type)	I and II	2	5
	III	3	
Schizophrenic reaction (schizoaffective type)	I and II	1	1
Nonpsychotics	I and II	5	5
Total		26	26

*Social classification used is based on the British Classification of Occupations (1950) as follows:

- Class I: Professional, etc; occupations: eg, doctors, professional engineers, accountants, commissioned officers
- Class II: Intermediate occupations: eg, industrial managers, business proprietors, pharmacists, costing clerks
- Class III: Skilled occupations: eg, joiners, electricians, plumbers
- Class IV: Partially skilled occupations: eg, farm laborers, railway firemen, bus conductors
- Class V: Unskilled occupations: eg, laborers, porters

It is important to note here that only one patient of the 26 had developed symptoms of confusion or delirium, and this was confirmed by the obstetricians and family physicians who first had seen the patients, prior to their admission to the psychiatric ward.

In our group, the appearance of the psychiatric symptoms took place between four and nine days postpartum. Furthermore, it was found that 12% in the schizophrenic group had a family history of mental illness, in contrast to 8% in the nonschizophrenic group. In addition, 50% in the schizophrenic group had a definite abnormal personality makeup (schizoid) in contrast to 26% in the nonschizophrenic group whose personality structure was suggestive of a mixed type of character disorder.

None of the patients in either group gave a history of a mental illness associated with a previous parturition (average number of pregnancies was three).

From the socioeconomic point of view, it is important to note here that of the 16 patients of the schizophrenic group, six belonged to the I and II social class (see Table 14-1), five to the III social class, and five to the IV and V social class. Of the five patients of the manic-depressive group, two belonged to the I and II social class and three to the III social class. Of the five patients of the neurotic group, all of them belonged to the I and II social class.

CASE HISTORY

The salutary effect of our therapeutic regime upon hospitalized patients suffering from a postpartum psychiatric syndrome will be shown in the following case history.

The patient, 22 years of age, was married in 1958 to a farmer six years her senior. She had two children, three and two years old.

The patient was admitted to the Provincial Mental Hospital on May 18, 1962, nine days postpartum.

Life Situation

Parents Mother had died at the age of 30 from postpartum hemorrhage when patient was 1½ years old. Her father was remarried when she was 8 years old. There was no evidence to suggest conflicts with her parents, in fact, she described both the father and the stepmother as "wonderful people."

Basic personality She was a very inadequate type of person having, at the same time, a profound "inferiority complex" due to her physique (obese).

Marital life—husband She described him as being withdrawn and unsociable. In general, she felt unhappy.

Social relations—adaptability She did not have close friends and felt rejected by the few with whom she made an attempt to relate. A great deal of anxiety and "shame" were present in her interpersonal relationships, particularly when the husband was with her.

Pregnancy Her feelings at the beginning of the pregnancy were acceptance of it, but later on, she developed anxiety and fear, for she felt inadequate to confront the new responsibilities.

Labor—delivery During the labor period, she was rather calm and the delivery was normal; a baby of seven pounds was born under general anesthesia.

Day of Crisis

This began immediately following her discharge from the hospital (sixth post delivery day). Thus, upon her arrival at home she started to talk to her older children, assuring them that "I love you . . . you both are members of the family." On the same day she became depressed, confused and, having the baby in her arms, she went back to the hospital where she began to scream "I am going to die." She was taken home, and the next day she felt absolutely inadequate and incapable of taking care of the baby. In view of these feelings, she called upon a relative to assist her and, in particular, to bathe the baby. While the relative was still at her home, she developed a psychotic reaction accompanied by somatic delusions (she thought that all her blood had left her body and that the placenta was still inside of her).

On the ninth postpartum day, her condition because worse, and she attempted to kill herself (threw herself out of the first floor window and was injured in the face).

Initial Interview

During the initial session, the patient was very apathetic and preoccupied with suicidal ideas and thoughts. Furthermore, she was extremely melancholic and considered herself a very inadequate person. In addition, feelings of guilt and futility were present, accompanied by auditory hallucinations, paranoid ideas, and self-accusations. Her affect was inappropriate and her insight into her illness nil. Both memory and orientation were intact in all spheres.

Diagnosis

Acute schizophrenic reactions (schizoaffective type).

Treatment—Progress

Her physical condition was within normal limits, and all the laboratory tests revealed no abnormality, including PBI. Thorazine, 75 mg qid, in combination with Elavil, 25 mg tid, was given and her condition was improving considerably.

Unfortunately, on June 17, 1962, one month following her admission to the hospital, she again developed paranoid ideas, delusions accompanied by profound depression, and suicidal ideas. In view of these developments, we administered electroconvulsive therapy (ECT) twice a week, along with the above-mentioned regime. She received a full course of 21 ECTs and was discharged on August 30, 1962, free of any psychotic symptoms, having made at the same time a satisfactory psychological and social recovery.

DISCUSSION

The very complicated thesis of the postpartum psychiatric syndromes is still in the stage of investigation.

In our opinion, special research teams (obstetricians–gynecologists, psychiatrists, psychologists, biochemists, etc) should investigate more thoroughly these syndromes under the prism of a psychophysiological approach.

Furthermore, we believe that the type of postpartum psychiatric illness depends to a great degree upon the basic personality structure of the woman prior to her illness.

SUMMARY

This study reports 26 patients who have been treated for postpartum psychiatric syndromes. The following observations were made:

1. Of these 26, 15 were schizophrenics (paranoid type), five were suffering from a manic-depressive psychosis, five were found to be nonpsychotics, and one was suffering from schizoaffective psychosis.
2. Of 26, none had developed delirium, and only one became confused during the acute episode.
3. The development of the different psychiatric symptoms occurred between four and nine days postpartum.
4. The combination of ECT, Thorazine, and Elavil (Destounis, 1956) gave us excellent therapeutic results.
5. From our studies and continuous investigations, we do not hesitate to suggest that the problem of postpartum psychiatric syndromes should be approached psychosociophysiologically.

CHAPTER 15

SEVERE PSYCHOLOGIC DISORDERS OF THE PUERPERIUM. A Recommended Approach for the Clinical Obstetrician

JOHN M. ASTRACHAN

This report presents a study of a group of women who manifested profound psychologic upheavals after childbirth. Further, it provides an approach and a way of organizing data that will better enable the psychologically minded obstetrician to anticipate possible postpartum emotional disturbance in his patients. Since the discussion is directed primarily to the clinical obstetrician, detailed consideration of the psychodynamics and the treatment of these women was excluded. In the commentary, a formulation is offered which will both aid in broadening understanding of these problems and suggest their pathogenesis.

MATERIAL AND METHOD

Thirteen patients comprised the study group. Twelve were studied subsequent to their admission to the psychiatric inpatient service of the Bronx Municipal Hospital Center. One woman, seen as an outpatient at the same institution, was evaluated in four extensive interviews preparatory to entering into long-term clinical psychotherapy. All hospitalized patients were evaluated, observed, and treated by the author during his psychiatric residency training under the supervision of senior staff psychiatrists.

A detailed study of each case was accomplished. Retrospective observations were then made as if the patient were being "seen" in the antepartum phase of her pregnancy and then in the postpartum period. The antepartum observations were then grouped. The same was done in the postpartum phase.

THE OBSTETRICIAN AS OBSERVER OF PSYCHOLOGIC DISORDERS

It is well known that the pregnant woman tends to exhibit a host of varying psychologic portraits. Most practicing obstetricians know this and are concerned with the psychologic aspects of their patients. Explanation, "talking to," and reassurance have long been measures accepted and utilized by the obstetric community in dealing with the sensitive psyche of the pregnant woman. There is little question that these approaches have added appreciably to the comfort and well-being of many patients. The physician, assuming the role of the kind, concerned imparter of information and dispeller of ignorance and fear, also obtains satisfaction. However, these measures provide no real understanding as to why the patient behaves as she does and develops, for example, a postpartum emotional disturbance.

The psychologically minded obstetrician uses supportive and educational techniques when needed. However, he differs from his reassuring and explaining confreres by adding an assiduously applied method of data collection to his procedure. The same painstaking care used in the evaluation of his patient's physical condition must be applied in his attempt to assess her psychologic state.

Several sources of information are available to the obstetrician. The referring physician may have information concerning medical complications treated, the patient's personal life and background, the family reaction to illness, and the type of people involved and their life situation.

Secondly, the people who accompany the patient to the office may further round out the picture of the patient's milieu. For example, are they anxious, angry, impatient, depressed, demanding, resentful, or passive? The interaction between the patient and the person accompanying her during the interview may provide clues. Again, if the patient's companion is amenable to it, inquiry about his or her concern over the pregnancy and any personal knowledge of the patient may yield useful information.

Thirdly, the office nurse may be a good source of information. She must be made to understand that the physician's interest in what she "knows" about a patient stems solely from his desire to attain a higher level of patient care. The nurse may also act as a "control" for the doctor, ie, her response to the individual patient could be compared to her previous responses to others.

The patient herself is the prime source of data. Collection of information of all kinds is the *sine qua non* of the psychologically minded obstetrician. Observation of the patient's general interest in her pregnancy, her response to physical changes, the quality and quantity of her complaints, and her appearance and demeanor is essential. During her labor, delivery, and hospital stay, the same constant observations should prevail.

ANTEPARTUM OBSERVATION

In the cases under study, it was thought that the most significant information relevant to the patient's eventual postpartum behavior might be obtained by concentrated inquiry into three areas: (1) past history of mental disease; (2) the relationship of the patient with her mother; (3) the relationship of the patient with her father.

Past History of Mental Disease

A history of emotional disturbance will naturally alert the clinician to the possibility of an exacerbation during or after pregnancy. However, such information will not always be easily obtainable, unless specifically sought. A routine "first-visit" question regarding past hospitalizations might be interpreted by the patient as referable only to physical illnesses. Furthermore, even if asked specifically about psychiatric hospitalizations, many patients will deny or evade the question, in an attempt to confine the obstetrician to his specialty. It is important to understand why this happens.

What the patient tells the obstetrician is a function of the type of relationship that she has with him. So-called "good rapport" is crucial and is dependent on the characteristics of both doctor and patient. Of importance is the general image that the obstetrician has in this country. To risk a generalization, the obstetrician is associated with predominantly pleasant things: new bouncing babies, family celebrations, listening to the fetal heart for the first time and being thrilled by it, fashionable maternity clothes and, in this day, almost a guarantee of good fetal and maternal results. He is thought of as a doctor for the "unsick." Further, in many communities, the woman's selection of the obstetrician is decreed in much the same way as is the choice of hairdresser, ie, the current vogue. The happy "image," on occasion, is extended until the obstetrician is seen as a symbol of normality, epitomizing societal restrictions to the patient. As a result, the patient does not discuss thorny items, such as hospitalization for mental illness, with her doctor.

Even under optimum conditions, some patients may not detail their difficulties. This is true, in the main, of the psychotic group. One patient in the series said she dared not tell her physician about her past psychiatric history for fear that discussing it might in some way make it return. Another patient reported, while she was extremely disorganized, that she was afraid to talk to her obstetrician for fear he would catch her difficulties from her, "like measles or something." The same patient said that she felt easier with a psychiatrist because he was "used to people like me." One useful hint to the obstetrician with respect to borderline or psychotic patients is to heed his own "feeling" about the patient. These are valid data which may manifest themselves in innumerable ways, depending on the obstetrician's own psychologically tender areas. In general, a sense of disquiet or discomfort coupled with a feeling of strangeness or unfamiliarity are good clues for the obstetrician to follow up.

In the series, with regard to a past history of emotional illness, patients were categorized as follows: (1) those having a history of psychiatric institutionalization (cases D, K, and L); (2) those treated psychiatrically in the past but not institutionalized (cases B, C, and E); and (3) those having no contact with a psychiatrist, yet manifesting behavior indicating that their handling of stress situations was in some way notably compromised. Aside from the difficulties described, it is relatively easy for the active interrogator to obtain information from the first two groups.

In the third group, however, the situation is less clear. Here the disturbance has been untreated or forgotten, or it has been categorized as a "normal human reaction" by the force of the patient's denial. This group of patients is the most taxing to the physician seeking significant psychologic material, because he must make a qualitative assessment of a sometimes single response. However, an attempt should be made to search the patient's deep feelings. In the study cases, probing the patient's response to great loss, shock, and anger provided the most revealing information. Inquiry can be made through a direct question. For example, what personal loss was the hardest for you to take in your life and what did you do when it happened? Although all the patients in the study group revealed some retrospective evidence of compromise in their reactions to stress, the two reported below seemed particularly suited to serve as examples of this group.

Case A The patient was admitted with an acute schizophrenic episode after birth of her first child. Her behavioral aberration amazed her family and obstetrician, as she had seemed so "normal" before the psychotic episode. She had graduated from high school, had a responsible job, and was supposedly happily married. Her obstetrician testified to her cheerful and cooperative manner and to the lack of any nervousness. During her restitutive phase in the hospital, the patient reported that at age 15 she was living with her mother's current boy friend, an alcoholic, and having intercourse with him intermittently after he had seduced her. One night he entered her room, told her to take care of her mother, went into the bathroom, and shot himself through the mouth. For a week after this understandably shocking experience the patient could not tell who she was or what had happened. This response under stress has an implication to the observer different from, for example, an extended crying spell.

Case G The patient was admitted following a suicide attempt. During treatment, she told of her reaction to the death of her fiancé in the war when she was 24 years old. Upon hearing the news she had immediately found herself unable to "do anything." This lasted for a year and included a great difficulty in leaving her home during that time.

Relationship with the Mother

In the psychologic evaluation of the pregnant patient, this area, crucial in the psychologic estimation of any person, assumes an even greater relative importance.

First, the new mother is confronted by the task of "mothering" an infant unable to care for itself for a long time. Also, the infant gives relatively little to the mother, while its demands are incessant. Complicating this already difficult situation is the special stress imposed by childbirth which induces in almost every woman deep concern over being cared for in a primitive oral sense. As Benedek (1949) put it: "There is an identification of the mother with the child which is interchangeable and is expressed actively as a wish to nurse and feed, and at the same time to be fed and cared for passively."

Although numerous factors may influence the parturient in either direction, the prime determinants of her behavior are the recollections, conscious and unconscious, of the "mothering" that she herself had received. Thus it was felt that a detailed investigation was needed of the relationship of the emotionally disturbed postpartum patient to her mother, especially from the standpoint of the patient's mother's capacity to gratify the patient's dependency need.

In 12 patients in the series, three significant events were discovered in the lives of their mothers which undoubtedly adversely affected the quality of "mothering" available to these women. These past disturbances were revivified by the patients in relating to their newborns and involved (1) the presence of serious maternal psychopathology, with (cases B, C, and K) and without (cases A, D, H, and L) a past history of maternal hospitalization; (2) death of the mother (cases G, I, and J); and (3) divorce in the family (cases E, F, and J).

Division of those mothers hospitalized and not hospitalized is important only from the standpoint of obtaining the information regarding the presence of maternal psychopathology. Obviously, it is easier to make the diagnosis of severe psychopathology if the patient was hospitalized. Furthermore, the hospitalization itself is only cogent in that the daughters of these disturbed women were exposed continuously to the degree of psychopathology which eventually necessitated hospitalization.

Although it did not occur in the study cases, the importance of the death of mother surrogates should be mentioned. This is especially true in cultures where grandmothers or aunts customarily take over much of the mothering function from the real mother. Under these circumstances, the death may have the same significance psychologically as the death of the real mother.

With respect to a divorce in the family, it is important to be aware that, although the divorce itself undoubtedly has great meaning to the mother, the situation between the parents preceding the divorce and its effect on the mother were the chief eventual pathogens for the patient.

Relationship with the Father

With the discovery that basic need-gratification patterns were generally distorted in this group of patients in their interaction with their mothers, an investigation of the relation to the other crucial family member—the father—was undertaken.

Significant circumstances obtaining with respect to the father were (1) his absence and (2) overt psychopathology on his part. With respect to absence, this could be: (1) absolute through death (cases C, H, and L); (2) absolute through physical separation (cases A, E, F, J, and I); and (3) relative, because of father's lack of "presence." In cases D, K, and B, conditions were similar. These men stayed with their families, but all were married to highly disturbed women and used avoidance as their method of dealing with the situation. All kept themselves overbusy in their lives outside the family and had little contact with the patients.

A striking feature in these patients was the vagueness of the relationship with their fathers even when the latter were present. In most instances, the father was absent. However, in those cases in which he was present and in reasonably good mental health, the patients made little mention of him. There could be many reasons for this; noteworthy, however, was the highly charged relationship of the patient with her mother which caused the father to be little more than a shadowy figure.

Implicit in the findings on the relationship of the patients to their fathers is again a significant lack of basic need fulfillment.

POSTPARTUM OBSERVATIONS

In this phase of contact with his patient, the obstetrician is somewhat hindered in his ability to collect psychologic data. Chiefly, this difficulty is due to the patient's abrupt cessation of frequent visits after delivery. However, observations can be made immediately after delivery, during the usual hospital visits, and at the six-week and six-month checkups. During this time, the clinician's most important communication with his patient is via the telephone, and a call may be the only clue available to the doctor as to the onset of a disturbance. It is probably safe to say that following the patient's discharge from the hospital, many obstetricians tend to feel that their job has been completed. But postpartum disturbances occur just at this point: that is, when the physician is no longer seeing the patient, when she has been discharged from the hospital, and the doctor is "relaxed." This discrepancy between the immediate emotional needs of the troubled patient and the psychologic unavailability of the obstetrician requires comment. The basic question is how far the responsibility of the obstetrician extends. It is clear from the cases under study that this responsibility must extend past the discharge from the hospital since the obstetrician is the professional person who has been in charge of the patient's welfare for nine months. The patient naturally will call upon him in her hour of difficulty. He must be available, and the patient must feel that he is.

The form in which an emotional disturbance appears after childbirth will obviously depend, as it does at any time in a person's life, on the specific psychodynamics of the individual concerned. The question is whether any aspects of woman's postpartum behavior might serve the obstetrician in evaluating an individual case. The answer is that there exists a near-universal behavior pattern observable within the first few months after delivery. This near-common denominator is usually referred to as "baby blues." More scientifically this phenomenon is termed "a tendency toward regression." Since this tendency is present to different degrees in all puerperal women, of critical importance is its extent. The women in this study all exhibited significant degrees of regression; superimposed were the specific individual psychodynamics which made for the differences in clinical status.

If the obstetrician knows the characteristics of the regressed patient, what fosters regression, and what constitutes highly regressive behavior, he will better understand a basic feature of psychology of the puerperal woman.

In a recent study of the psychology of pregnancy, this definition of regression was provided (Bibring, 1961):

> A return to an earlier stage of functioning in order to avoid the anxieties and hostilities involved in later stages; a reestablishment of an earlier stage where conflict was less. As a purposive way of handling a specific conflictual situation, regression is a defense and an ego mechanism. It is a "way out" and, as it were, a flight into earlier modes of adjustment.

When a postpartum woman becomes regressed, her behavioral characteristics are usually those demonstrated by the child she has just delivered. She will show excessive mood lability with easy crying, hyperirritability, and, in general, a low tolerance for frustration. She will seem to be saying constantly, "I want what I want when I want it." Also, usually untroubled functions, such as sleep or eating, may be disturbed. Regressive behavior is certainly not confined to this period in the life of a woman; it can occur under varied circumstances. The fact to be emphasized is that in the postpartum patient, regression is to some degree practically omnipresent. When a patient shows this or tells about it, it must be evaluated as to its degree and not dismissed. Such evaluation requires sound clinical judgment. This can be attained by the obstetrician as are other clinical skills—by constant critical observations.

Society has evolved ways of helping the pregnant woman ward off "return to an earlier stage of functioning in order to avoid the anxieties and hostilities involved in later stages." These societal measures allow the woman to feel special and cared for and make "the later stages" as easy as possible. In this country, some examples include: canned baby foods, disposable bottles, diaper services, maternity fashion consultants, advice-to-mothers columns in magazines, decorative birth announcement cards, and presents of flowers and candy to the mother from friends and family. The obstetrician can be viewed as a sort of cultural medical outgrowth of the need for dealing in a "special" way with the "delicate" condition of the pregnant patient. Further, the accoutrements of obstetric practice, such as maternity hospitals, instruction classes, and much of prenatal care, add to the aura of "specialness" that surrounds the pregnant woman. As the societal representative of all of this supportive, antiregressive effort, the obstetrician feels tremendous pressure.

The supportive protection resulting from all these efforts will, in most instances, allow the patient to keep out of difficulty. However, the obstetrician must be prepared for other eventualities.

In the study cases, it became apparent that several events played a part in fostering severe regressions; these included physical illness in the baby or the mother, a rejecting husband, lack of supportive parents, economic difficulties, and the actions of the physician. Superimposed upon the damage to the lives of these women in years past, these served often as the straw that broke the camel's back.

Physical Illness in the Baby

Case H Three days after the patient's return from the hospital everything seemed to go wrong. The baby had feeding difficulties necessitating treatment, including formula changes, sedation, threatened and then canceled hospitalization for the child, numerous visits to pediatricians' offices, and a difficult feeding schedule. The patient became more and more distraught and began to feel as if the baby was the whole problem: "I would wake up tense as a board, and during the day would get blackouts and dizzy spells." She found herself shaking when she had to pick up her child. However, she acknowledged that the baby probably was not to blame, as she recalled that all of her adult life she had felt a virtual inability to be around children less than eight months old. The patient was admitted after attempting to kill herself.

In such cases the obstetrician sometimes can play an important role. A feeding problem may not only be symptomatic of pyloric stenosis but may also indicate a pathologic mother–child relationship.

A rather common feature found in the study cases was the fear of these women that they would harm the baby. Childbirth does not always engender feelings of loving motherliness in the woman. Seeds of ambivalence toward the child are present to some degree in each mother, since her maternal attitudes are colored by her past experience with her own mother. This is often at the root of the common fear of hurting the baby.

In most of the women, even having an idea of a hostile impulse to the child produced intolerable guilt feelings and profound psychic discomfort. However, the expression of such thoughts often prompted the patient's family or the obstetrician to initiate psychiatric treatment.

Physical Illness in the Mother

Obviously many "sick" patients in the hospital show signs of regressive behavior, often call "hospitalitis." In the study series, there were four cases involving significant obstetric complications. Case C was that of a patient with severe postpartum hemorrhage followed by pyelonephritis. After the latter was under control, she developed an acute demyelinating disease. In case G an elderly primigravida had a long, difficult labor with a postpartum hemorrhage. In case H the patient had a postpartum hemorrhage, and in case J, long, painful, difficult labor was followed by a grossly infected episiotomy and endometritis.

Furthermore, two others had complications of a less acute nature. Nevertheless, considering the fact that one (case D) had no prenatal care and the other (case L) suffered from severe weight loss in the first trimester of pregnancy which repeated itself postpartum, these difficulties conceivably contributed to the development of the postpartum disturbances in these women.

Presence of a Rejecting Husband

A rejecting husband was a factor in cases A, F, G, I, and J. In these cases, the spectrum of husband behavior varied from overt rejection to subtle nonsupportiveness. The following demonstrates how, in a sensitive situation, such a circumstance can add fuel to the fire.

Case J The patient's husband related that two months prior to marriage, his wife and he had had intercourse and that it had been hard for her. However, he said, he "always knew when a woman was crazy about him" and connected this with the fact that she "didn't make a fuss about it." He added that sometimes he would tease her by saying that he would not marry her, to which she would respond, "Whatever you want is all right with me." He revealed further that he had never told her that he loved her, "because I liked her the way she was and I didn't want to spoil her." He continued that he usually stayed away from home in the evening until 3 or 4 AM, spending his time in a neighborhood bar, but he denied going with other women. During her hospital stay, the patient bitterly complained about her husband's practice of coming to see her five minutes before the end of visiting hours. Because of this she felt that he did not care about her.

Lack of Supportive Parents

Most women have a special need for support and nurturing by their parents at this time. In the study group, it was evident that the relative unavailability of parents to gratify the needs of these patients resulted in furthering their regressive trends. In general, when people of significance are absent, dead, in a different country, or too ill themselves to render support, the new mother suffers greatly. In each case in the study group, this deficiency existed.

For example, in case G, the patient's mother had died in childbirth and her father was in Germany. The patient's sister lived at a distance and was relatively unavailable. It is of significance that in two patients (cases L and G), admission for psychiatric care followed upon the departure of the baby nurses, both of whom were motherly figures. The absence of supportive people, or the patient's dismissal from a supportive, need-gratifying place like the hospital may tend often to aggravate an already trying situation.

Case K shows how the obstetrician may become involved in a need-gratifying sense, especially when other sources are not available. In practice, these are the patients with whom the clinician may become annoyed; they are the "complainers."

Case K In the initial psychiatric hospital interview, the patient stated:

> My labor was induced—he stopped it so that he could get back to his office for hours. He also sent me home too quickly because my stitches were still hurting—besides, I had a bad hemorrhoid. He gave me no breast pills or vitamins to take home, he let my labor go on too long, and didn't talk to me after the delivery. He's a butcher and charged me too much—the needles that he gave me hurt too much and didn't do a thing for my pain. He shouldn't be doing obstetrics, and I want you [the examiner] to help me sue him. I was pretty good in the hospital, but as soon as I walked out and into my house the trouble started. My father manages a supermarket—do you think he filled the refrigerator or anything; do you think that anyone did anything for me at all?

Throughout her statement, we can see the patient's rage at her doctor; however, we can also see the basic reason for it. She juxtaposed her comments about the obstetrician with those about her father's failure to feed her. So, basically, she is crying out because she felt deprived in a primitive oral sense. It is easy to become annoyed with such a patient, but so much better to find out what her anger is really about and how it is being transferred to the physician in the case. (It is of interest that in this case the mother was a highly disorganized, chronic schizophrenic, unable to render any useful support.)

Economic Difficulties

All the women studied were clinic patients, implying that their financial resources were limited. However, in most instances the husbands worked regularly and usually managed fairly well. Only in case F did financial insecurity play a significant role. This patient was completely on her own resources. She had no family, was not legally married, and was completely dependent on the man with whom she lived. His threat to withdraw what meager support he did offer unless she gave up the baby added to her difficulties.

Actions of the Physician

Three study patients (cases G, H, and M) were admitted to the hospital following suicide attempts. All used the medication given by the obstetrician to "relax" them. In each instance, they had telephoned the physician, who had then ordered "a little sedation" by telephone. One woman was advised to take a trip. All were reassured that women have a little trouble sleeping after delivery and that they would be all right.

Case J This patient complained to the obstetrician of weeping and irritability. By telephone, he prescribed Compazine (25 mg every 12 hours). When it was not successful, he recommended that the patient visit an internist, who diagnosed a "postpartum psychosis" and doubled the dosage of Compazine. This was also unsuccessful, and finally the husband took the patient to a local hospital where psychiatric hospitalization was advised. At admission the patient was in a state of complete confusion, rigid, and drooling from Compazine toxicity. There was little doubt that the medication had potentiated her psychologic difficulty.

It is not accidental that the patients who attempted suicide did so by taking something given them by their doctor to put in their mouths and make them feel better. It has been repeatedly emphasized in this paper how prominent the oral-dependent-regressive pattern is in the pregnant patient. It was almost as if these women were trying to feed on and incorporate within themselves the part of the giving doctor for whom they had such great need. In short, "a little sedation" at a distance and unsupervised is a dangerous thing, since the medical use of tranquilizers, although often effective, is just as often perverted by the need of the regressed patient. In these cases close supervision is an absolute necessity.

Most important in the cases noted above is the attitudes of the physicians involved. Their denial of the symptom picture presented by these patients was operative. The fact that the patients attempted suicide points up the danger of denial by the doctor.

COMMENT

A tendency toward regressive behavior is an almost universal finding in the puerperal woman. It is certainly true of the disturbed patient. Further, in the postpartum period, physiologic changes of large magnitude are known to occur (Bower and Altschule, 1956). Since regressive behavior is so common at this time, one may logically assume that it might be the psychologic reflection of the ongoing biologic processes.

Also, it seems conceivable that even in a psychologically "normal" postpartum woman some psychologic manifestation of the biologic process might exist. An illuminating interview with a psychologist who had recently given birth and who could be considered "normal" comes closest to indicating what the psychological manifestations might be. Just prior to nursing her baby, she would experience a depression lasting for half a minute, associated with a feeling of imminent depletion. This would pass before the nursing began but was of such intensity that she was conscious of real discomfort. She told of no associated thought with the sensation and reported: "It just seemed to happen all of a sudden." Her general puerperal behavior was characterized by mild mood changes.

Combining impressions obtained from analysis of the study patients with the considerations above enables us to indicate a tentative formulation for the pathogenesis of the puerperal psychologic disorders. It may be theorized that each puerperal woman experiences feelings of depression and depletion, coupled with a tendency towards regression. These feelings probably reflect the physiologic changes at this time and may be considered the psychologic "baseline" of general postpartum behavior. The experimental variables present in the individual woman will influence the development and outcome of such feelings.

In a group of sorely disturbed patients whose behavior departed from the "baseline," three main areas were investigated:

1. The relationship of the patient to her mother. It was discovered that in a majority (12), events were found in the lives of their mothers that resulted in a faulty "mothering" experience for the patients. These occurrences were death of the mother, divorce in the family, or severe maternal psychopathology.

2. The relationship of the patient to her father. Investigation revealed the majority (11) to have fathers who were absent to varying

degrees, as a result of death, physical separation, or "lack of presence." The remainder (two) had fathers who showed significant psychopathology.

3. Factors promoting regression especially operative and damaging in the postpartum period. These include illness in the mother, illness in the baby, a rejecting husband, absence of supportive family members, socioeconomic factors, and iatrogenic factors.

These features, with the exception of the postpartum factors, were seen to have had a deleterious effect on several of the patients before their puerperal breakdown. It was notable that six had received prior psychiatric aid, either as inpatients (three) or outpatients (three). There was retrospective evidence in the others (seven) that there was a serious deficiency in their ability to withstand stress situations (Table 15-1).

It should be pointed out that although the family data are suggestive, no cause-and-effect relationship is implied. It is understandable that a woman who had a chronic schizophrenic mother and a father who abandoned her and who herself was institutionalized at adolescence is likely to have trouble after childbirth. However, it may not hold true, and the most likely candidate for trouble may have learned modes of defense in the course of her adaptation that will enable her to get by without appreciable difficulty.

It is anticipated that a study will be conducted to compare the familial situations of patients with psychologically "normal" puerperiums to those who experience difficulties. Further, the formulation that has been offered requires testing in an anterospective fashion, and data must be collected. Of interest would be the evaluation (in terms of regressive responses) of women who adopt newborn children.

With regard to the obstetrician's management of an individual case, three courses of action are open: investigation, treatment, or referral.

Investigation

It has been emphasized that investigation and data collection are of great importance in approaching these problems. Other factors operate which increase the difficulty in accomplishing this objective and involve the obstetrician and his attitudes.

First, the complaint is often voiced of the time limitations implicit in obstetric practice. A routine case requires approximately 10–11 hours. Admission procedures at most psychiatric clinics consume about half that time. Clearly the question is not the amount of time available but how that time is utilized.

Secondly, practitioners will complain that the practice of obstetrics is hard enough without adding the burden of personal anxieties, which are stirred up by contact with disturbed patients. There is no doubt that

Table 15-1
Data on Patients Manifesting Psychological Disorders after Childbirth

Case	Age	Race*	Religion†	Parity	Sex of Last Child	Admission Diagnosis
A	20	N	C	1	F	Acute paranoid schizophrenia
B	30	W	J	1	F	Chronic paranoid schizophrenia
C	25	W	J	1	F	Acute psychosis due to organic brain syndrome
D	34	W	J	3	M	Chronic paranoid schizophrenia
E	22	PR	C	2	F	Acute paranoid schizophrenia
F	34	N	C	2	M	Paranoid reaction with depression
G	40	W	C	1	F	Suicide attempt; depressive reaction
H	29	W	C	2	F	Suicide attempt; depressive reaction
I	27	N	C	2	M	Acute paranoid schizophrenia; Compazine toxicity
J	23	PR	C	2	F	Acute paranoid schizophrenia and depression
K	26	W	J	2	M	Manic phase of manic-depressive psychosis
L	23	W	J	1	F	Masochistic character disorder with depressive features
M	30	W	C	3	F	Depressive reaction; suicide attempt

*N = negro; W = white; PR = Puerto Rican.
†C = Catholic; J = Jewish.

Past History of Mental Disease	Relationship with Mother	Relationship with Father	Regressogenic Factors
No contact with psychiatrist; evidence of compromise in handling of stress situations	Divorce in family; mother disturbed; no hospitalization	Absolute absence due to physical separation	Rejecting husband; lack of supportive parents
Treated by psychiatrist; not hospitalized	Mother disturbed; hospitalized	Absence relative because of father's "lack of presence"	Lack of supportive parents
Treated by psychiatrist; not hospitalized	Mother disturbed; hospitalized	Absolute absence due to death of father	Physical illness in mother; lack of supportive parents
Hospitalized for psychiatric treatment	Mother disturbed; not hospitalized	Absence relative because of father's "lack of presence"	No husband; lack of supportive parents
Treated by psychiatrist; not hospitalized	Divorce in family	Absolute absence due to physical separation	Lack of supportive parents
No contact with psychiatrist; evidence of compromise in handling of stress situations	Divorce in family	Absolute absence due to physical separation	Rejecting husband; lack of supportive parents; socioeconomic factors
No contact with psychiatrist; evidence of compromise in handling of stress situations	Death of mother	Father disturbed; not hospitalized or treated	Illness of mother; lack of supportive parents; rejecting husband; iatrogenic factors
No contact with psychiatrist; evidence of compromise in handling of stress situations	Mother disturbed; not hospitalized	Absolute absence due to death of father	Illness of mother; illness of baby; absence of supportive parents; iatrogenic factors
No contact with psychiatrist; evidence of compromise in handling of stress situations	Death of mother	Absolute absence due to physical separation	Rejecting husband; lack of parents; iatrogenic factors
No contact with psychiatrist; evidence of compromise in handling of stress situations	Death of mother; divorce in family	Absolute absence due to physical separation	Illness of mother; lack of parents; rejecting husband
Hospitalized for psychiatric treatment	Mother disturbed; hospitalized	Relative absence due to "lack of presence"	Lack of supportive parents
Hospitalized for psychiatric treatment	Mother disturbed; not hospitalized	Absolute absence due to death of father	Illness of mother; lack of parental support
No contact with psychiatrist; evidence of compromise in handling of stress situations		Father disturbed; not hospitalized or treated	Iatrogenic factors

merely attempting to observe a disturbed patient is a trying and sometimes enervating experience. However, the obstetrician can try to keep the patient's behavior under objective scrutiny. Further, the obstetrician who has had the benefits of psychoanalysis can be more at ease in his interaction with patients in general and disturbed ones in particular.

Treatment

One reward of obstetrical practice is, in most instances, the ability of the physician to do something for his patient. Many obstetricians have difficulty appreciating that in dealing with the psychologic aspects of their patients, they need not do anything actively to be of appreciable aid. A kindly, nonjudgmental, objective, data-collecting approach, when combined with the patient's confidence in the skill, integrity, and gentleness of the physician, will help her. It will also allow the doctor to be knowledgeable about her in depth.

If the obstetrician finds factors in the patient's family that might predispose her to trouble, he should be especially alert for the occurrence of factors which promote regression. This requires observation. One possible step is to see the "susceptible" patient more than just at her six-week checkup. The dependence of the woman on her obstetrician would thus have a chance to subside more gently than is the usual case. These may appear to be rather simple measures, but to a disturbed patient an audience with an objective, sympathetic person may be most helpful.

Referral to a Psychiatrist

Ideally, a psychiatric referral should mean no more to a patient than a consultation with another specialist. In the study cases, patient resistance was not the key factor, although it played a part. To no patient in the series was the suggestion made that she see a psychiatrist, even where previous psychiatric hospitalization was a part of the history. There is no question that with a past history of psychiatric care, referral for a current evaluation is in order.

What about the patient whose problems fall into the categories noted? The possibilities for combinations are endless. For example, does a patient whose mother had two visits with a psychiatrist after the death of her husband require referral? Does one whose father died when she was 9 years old? The ultimate decision in each instance must be made by the obstetrician after he obtains adequate information. Further, he must have available psychiatric colleagues with whom he may discuss questionable cases. This free interchange between the psychiatrist and the obstetrician must be sought and fostered by each specialist.

SUMMARY

Thirteen women presenting with severe psychologic disturbances in the puerperium were studied. Emphasizing concerns of importance to the clinical obstetrician, this study provides an approach to these disorders which will help the obstetrician in dealing with these situations.

A tentative formulation is offered with regard to the pathogenesis of emotional disturbances occurring in the puerperium.

BIBLIOGRAPHY

American Psychiatric Association: *Diagnostic and Statistical Manual of Mental Disorders*, 3rd ed. Washington, DC, APA, 1980.

Anderson EW: Psychiatric aspects of abortion. Proceedings of the Third World Congress of Psychiatry, Montreal, Canada, June 4–10, 1961. Toronto, University of Toronto Press, 1961, Vol II, pp 1170–1174.

Arén P, Åmark C: Prognosen vid beviljad men icke utförd legal abort. *Sven Läkartidn* 1957;54:3709.

Arthure H: Suicide in pregnancy. *Br Med J* 1968;1:638.

Asch SS: Psychiatric complications, in Rovinsky JJ, Guttmacher AF (eds): *Medical, Surgical, and Gynecological Complications of Pregnancy*, 2nd ed. Baltimore, Williams & Wilkins, 1965, pp 461–472.

Asling J, Way EL: Placental transfer of drugs, in Ladu BN, Mandel HG, Way EL (eds): *Fundamentals of Drug Metabolism and Drug Disposition*. Baltimore, Williams & Wilkins, 1971, pp 88–102.

Assembly Bills No. 2614 and No. 2310, California Legislature, 1961. Regular session. Introduced by Mr. Knox and Mr. Beilenson, respectively.

Atkinson MW, Kessel N, Dalgaard JB: The comparability of suicide rates. *Br J Psychiatry* 1975;127:247–256.

Bardon D: Psychological implications of provision for childbirth. *Lancet* 1973; 2:555–558.

Barno A: Criminal abortion deaths, illegitimate pregnancy deaths, and suicides in pregnancy. Minnesota, 1950–1965. *Am J Obstet Gynecol* 1967;98:356–367.

Barraclough BM: Differences between national suicide rates. *Br J Psychiatry* 1973;122:95–96.

Barraclough BM: Scottish and English suicide rates. *Br J Psychiatry* 1974; 124:105–106.

Battle RJV, Marshall HES: Attempted suicide by burning. *Br Med J* 1952; 2:1397–1398.

deBeauvoir S: *The Second Sex*. New York, Knopf, 1968, pp 29–30.

Benedek T: The psychosomatic implications of the primary unit: Mother-child. *Am J Orthopsychiatry* 1949;19:642–654.

Benedek T: The psychobiology of pregnancy, in Anthony EJ, Benedek T (eds): *Parenthood*. Boston, Little, Brown & Company, 1970, pp 137–151.

Bengtsson L: Graviditet och självmord. *Sven Läkartidn* 1947;44:1469–1484.

Bertelsen A, Harvald B, Hauge M: A Danish twin study of manic-depressive disorders. *Br J Psychiatry* 1977;130:330–351.

Bibring GL: Some considerations of the psychological processes in pregnancy, *Psychoanal Study Child* 1959;14:113–121.

Bibring G: *Psychoanalytic Study of the Child*. New York, International University Press, 1961.

Bibring G, Valenstein AF: Biological aspects of pregnancy. *Clin Obstet Gynecol* 1976;19:357–371.

Binder H: Die psychiatrische Abortindikation. *Schweiz Med Wochenschr* 1943; 24:489; cited by Höök, 1963.

Binder H: Die psychiatrischen Indikationen zur Unterbrechung der Schwangerschaft. *Schweiz Arch Neurol Psychiat* 1951;67:245; cited by Höök, 1963.

Birtchnell J, Floyd S: Attempted suicide and the menstrual cycle – a negative conclusion. *J Psychosom Res* 1974;18:361–369.

Birtchnell J, Floyd S: Further menstrual characteristics of suicide attemptors. *J Psychosom Res* 1975;19:81–85.

Bolter S: The psychiatrist's role in therapeutic abortion: The unwitting accomplice. *Am J Psychiatry* 1962;119:312–316.

Bower WH, Altschule MD: Use of progesterone in the treatment of post-partum psychosis. *N Engl J Med* 1956;254:157–160.

Boxall JS, Chauvel PJ: Attempted suicide: A review of 100 consecutive cases at a district hospital. *Med J Aust* 1966;1:264–266.

Boyd DA Jr: Mental disorders associated with childbearing. *Am J Obstet Gynecol* 1942;43:335–348.

Braunstein GD, Rason J, Adler D, Danzer H, Wade ME: Serum human chorionic gonadotropin levels throughout normal pregnancy. *Am J Obstet Gynecol* 1976;126:678–681.

Braverman J, Roux JF: Screening for the patient at risk for postpartum depression. *Obstet Gynecol* 1978;52:731–736.

Brew MF, Seidenberg R: Reactions associated with pregnancy and childbearing. *J Nerv Ment Dis* 1950;11:408–423.

Brown GW, Harris T: *Social Origins of Depression.* London, Tavistock Publications, 1978.

Brown JH: Reporting of suicide: Canadian statistics. *Suicide Life Threat Behav* 1975;5:21–28.

Brown WA: *Psychological Care During Pregnancy and the Postpartum Period.* New York, Raven Press, 1979.

Browne WJ, Palmer AJ: A preliminary study of schizophrenic women who murdered their children. *Hosp Community Psychiatry* 1975;26:71–75.

Burke AW: Socio-cultural determinants of attempted suicide among West Indians in Birmingham: Ethnic origin and immigrant status. *Br J Psychiatry* 1976; 129:261–266.

Burke MF: Suicide in pregnancy. *Br Med J* 1968;2:49.

Butler JC, Reisner DP, Wagner NN: Sexuality during pregnancy and postpartum, in Green R (ed): *Human Sexuality – A Health Practitioner's Text.* Baltimore, Williams & Wilkins, 1979, pp 176–190.

California Penal Code, paragraph 274.

Carmen EH, Russo NF, Miller JB: Inequality and women's mental health. *Am J Psychiatry* 1981;38:1319–1330.

Chalupa M, Zdímalová M: Suicide of women with unwanted pregnancy. (*Excerpta Medica* 1969;2:15.) *Cs Gynek* 1968;33:608–610.

Chertok L: The psychopathology of vomiting of pregnancy, in Howells JG (ed): *Modern Perspectives in Psycho-obstetrics.* Edinburgh, Oliver & Boyd, 1972, p 269.

Cohen MB: Personal identity and sexual identity, in Miller JB (ed): *Psychoanalysis and Women.* New York, Brunner/Mazel, 1973, pp 131–155.

Cohler BJ, Gruenebaum HU, Weiss JL, Robbins DM, Schader RI, Gallant D, Hartman CR: Social role performance and psychopathology among recently hospitalized and non-hospitalized mothers. II. Correlates with life stress and self-reported psychopathology. *J Nerv Ment Dis* 1974;159:81–90.

Colman AD: Psychological state during first pregnancy. *Am J Orthopsychiatry* 1969;39:788–797.

Colman AD: Psychology of a first-baby group. *Int J Group Psychother* 1971; 21:74–83.

Dalton K: Menstruation and acute psychiatric illnesses. *Br Med J* 1959;1:148–149.

Dalton K: Menstruation and crime. *Br Med J* 1961;2:1752–1753.

Daly MJ: The emotional problems of patients encountered in the practice of obstetrics and gynecology. *Obstet Gynecol Annu* 1980;9:339–356.

Darkness at Noon. *New York Daily News*. March 23, 1983, p 4.

Daube D: The linguistics of suicide. *Suicide Life Threat Behav* 1977;7:132–182.

Destounis N: Electroshock in combination with muscular relaxants and oxygen. *J Méd Grèce* September 1, 1956.

Destounis N: Complications of pregnancy—a psychosomatic approach. *Can Psychiatr Assoc J* 1962;7:279–290.

Destounis N: The value of psychotherapy in pregnancy—a psychosomatic approach. Abstracts of the Sixth European Conference of Psychosomatic Research. Athens, Greece, May 6–9, 1964a.

Destounis N: Psychotherapy in pregnancy. Abstracts of the Sixth International Congress of Psychotherapy. London, England, August 24–29, 1964b.

Deutch H: *The Psychology of Women*, Vols 1 and 2. New York, Grune & Stratton, 1944–1945.

Donaldson JO: *Neurology of Pregnancy*. Philadelphia, WB Saunders, 1978, pp 251–262.

Doolittle J: *Social Life of the Chinese*. New York, Harper & Bros, 1865, vol 1, pp 108–110.

Douglas JD: *The Social Meaning of Suicide*. Princeton, Princeton University Press, 1967.

Dublin LI: *Suicide. A Sociological and Statistical Study*. New York, Ronald Press, 1963.

Durkheim E: *Suicide*. Glencoe, Illinois, Free Press, 1951 (originally published in 1897).

Ekblad M: Relation of the legal-abortion clientele to the illegal-abortion clientele and the risk of suicide. *Acta Psychiatr Neurol Scand* 1955a;Suppl 99:93–98.

Ekblad M: Induced abortion on psychiatric grounds. A follow-up study of 479 women. *Acta Psychiatr Neurol Scand* 1955b;Suppl 99:1–238.

Epps P: Women in prison on attempted suicide charges. *Lancet* 1957;2:182–184.

Ettlinger R: Evaluation of suicide prevention after attempted suicide. *Acta Psychiatr Scand* 1975;Suppl 260:1–135.

Eungprabhanth V: Suicide in Thailand. *Forensic Sci* 1975;5:43–51.

Evans JG: Deliberate self-poisoning in the Oxford area. *Br J Prev Soc Med* 1967; 21:97–107.

Fay E, Meskil P: Drowns baby in bathtub. *New York Daily News*. April 13, 1983, p 3.

Feggetter G: Suicide in opera. *Br J Psychiatry* 1980;136:552–557.

Firth R: Suicide and risk-taking in Tikopia society, in Giddens A (ed): *The Sociology of Suicide. A Selection of Readings*. London, Frank Cass, 1971, pp 197–222.

Fischer N: Multiple induced abortions. A psychoanalytic case study. *J Am Psychoanal Assoc* 1974;22:394–407.

Frederick CJ: Current trends in suicidal behavior in the United States. *Am J Psychother* 1978;32:172–200.

Freedman R, Whelpton P, Campbell A: *Family Planning, Sterility and Population Growth*. New York, McGraw-Hill, 1959, p 75.

Friedman E: The physiological aspects of pregnancy, in Notman MT, Nadelson CC (eds): *The Woman Patient*. New York, Plenum Press, 1978, pp 55–71.

Frommer EA, O'Shea G: Antenatal identification of women liable to have problems in managing their infants. *Br J Psychiatry* 1973;123:149–156.

Fuchs F, Klopper A: *Endocrinology of Pregnancy*. Hagerstown, Maryland, Harper & Row, 1976.

Gabrielson IW, Klerman LV, Currie JB, Tyler NC, Jekel JF: Suicide attempts in a population pregnant as teenagers. *Am J Public Health* 1970;60:2289–2301.

Gebhard PH, Pomeroy WB, Martin CE, Christenson CW: *Pregnancy, Birth and Abortion.* New York, Harper & Brothers and Paul B Hoeber, 1958, p 196.

Gelfand M: Suicide and attempted suicide in the urban and rural African in Rhodesia. *Cent Afr J Med* 1976;22:203–205.

General Statutes of Connecticut, Section 53-32, Revision of 1958.

Giddens A: *The Sociology of Suicide. A Selection of Readings.* London, Frank Cass, 1971.

Goldberg HL, DiMascio A: Psychotropic drugs in pregnancy, in Lipton MA, DiMascio LA (eds): *Psychopharmacology: A Generation of Progress.* New York, Raven Press, 1978, pp 1047–1055.

Golub MS, Golub AM: Behavioral teratogenesis, in Milunsky A, Friedman EA, Gluck L (eds): *Advances in Perinatal Medicine,* Vol 1. New York, Plenum Medical Book Company, 1981.

Goodhart CB: Suicide in pregnancy. *Br Med J* 1968;1:218.

Goodwin J: Suicide attempts in sexual abuse victims and their mothers. *Child Abuse Neglect* 1981;5:217–221.

Goodwin J, Harris D: Suicide in pregnancy: The Hedda Gabler syndrome. *Suicide Life Threat Behav* 1979;9:105–115.

Goodwin J, Jaramillo J: Postpartum psychosis in an artist. *Bull Birth Psychol* 1981;2:2–11.

Gordon M: *The Company of Women.* New York, Ballantine Books, 1980.

Gordon RE, Gordon KK: Social factors in the prediction and treatment of emotional disorders of pregnancy. *Am J Obstet Gynecol* 1959;77:1074–1083.

Gordon RE, Gordon KK: Social factors in prevention of postpartum emotional problems. *Obstet Gynecol* 1960;15:433–438.

Grimm ER: Psychological tension in pregnancy. *Psychosom Med* 1961;23:520–527.

Grimm ER, Gruenberg EM, Illsley R, et al: *Childbearing—Its Social and Psychological Aspects.* Richardson, SA, Guttmacher AF (eds). Baltimore, Williams & Wilkins, 1967.

Guernsey RS: *Suicide: History of the Penal Laws Relating to It in Their Legal, Social, Moral and Religious Aspects in Ancient and Modern Times.* New York, L.K. Strouse & Company, 1883.

Guttentag M, Salasin S, Belle D: *The Mental Health of Women.* New York, Academic Press, 1980.

Hamilton HA: *Postpartum Psychiatric Problems.* St. Louis, CV Mosby, 1962.

Harrington JA, Cross KW: Cases of attempted suicide admitted to a general hospital. *Br Med J* 1959;2:463–467.

Harvey D: Maternal mental illness—the effect on the baby, in Sandler M (ed): *Mental Illness in Pregnancy and the Puerperium.* New York, Oxford University Press, 1978, pp 112–119.

Hatherley LI, Breheny JE, Robinson FS, Beischer NA: Psychiatric disorders in obstetrics. *Med J Aust* 1979;2:399–401.

Hawes BL: LaLlorona in juvenile hall. *West Folklore* 1968;27:153–170.

Hay DM: Serum oestriol in normal pregnancy. *Br J Obstet Gynaecol* 1976;83:118–123.

Hayworth J, Little BC, Canten SB, Raptopoulos P, Priest RG, Sandler M: A predictive study of postpartum depressions—some predisposing characteristics. *Br J Med Psychol* 1980;53:161–167.

Heiman M: A psychoanalytic view of pregnancy, in Rovinsky JJ, Guttmacher AF (eds): *Medical, Surgical, and Gynecologic Complications of Pregnancy.* Baltimore, Williams & Wilkins, 1965.

Heller A, Whittington HG: The Colorado story: Denver General Hospital experience with the change in the law on therapeutic abortion. *Am J Psychiatry* 1968; 125:809–816.

Hirsh J: Suicide. Part 3: Dynamics of suicide. *Ment Hygiene* 1960;44:274–280.

Hirsh J: Cultural determinants of suicide. The perspective of the Japanese. *Ment Hyg* 1966;50:337–339.

Holmes ME, Klerman LV, Gabrielson IW: A new approach to educational services for pregnant students. *J Sch Health* 1970;40:168.

Höök K: Refused abortion. A follow-up study of 249 women whose applications were refused by the National Board of Health in Sweden. *Acta Psychiatr Scand* 1963;Suppl 168:1–156.

Höök K: Depression in unwanted children. Proceedings of the 4th UEP Congress, Stockholm, 1971, pp 116–125.

Höök K: The unwanted child-effects on mothers and children of refused applications for abortion, in Levy L (ed): *Society, Stress and Disease*, Vol 2. London, Oxford Medical Publications, 1975, pp 187–192.

Howard M: The Webster School. District of Columbia Program for Pregnant Girls. *U.S. Department of Health, Education and Welfare.* (Children's Bureau), Item 453-B, 1968.

Hultin M, Ottosson JO: Klinisk observation av abortsökande kvinnor. *Sven Läkartidn* 1962;59:1365.

Iga M, Yamamoto J, Noguchi T: The vulnerability of young Japanese women. *Suicide* 1975;5:207–222.

Inghe G: 1941 ars befolkningsutredning. Betänkande i abortfrågan (SOU 1944/51). Stockholm 1944; cited by Otto, 1965, p 284.

Jacobziner H: Attempted suicides in adolescence. *JAMA* 1965;191:101–105.

James IP, Derham SP, Scott-Orr DN: Attempted suicide—a study of 100 patients referred to a general hospital. *Med J Aust* 1963;50:375–380.

Jarrahi-Zadeh A, Kane FJ, VanDeCastle RL, Lachenbruch PA, Ewing JA: Emotional and cognitive changes in pregnancy and early puerperium. *Br J Psychiatry* 1969;115:797–805.

Jervis J: *On the Office and Duties of Coroners, with Forms and Precedents*, 9th ed. Purchase WB, Wollaston HW (eds). London, Sweet, 1957.

Jessner L, Weigert E, Foy, JL: The development of parental attitudes during pregnancy, in Anthony EJ (ed): *Parenthood: Its Psychology and Psychopathology.* Boston, Little, Brown, 1970, pp 209–244.

Jones A: *Women Who Kill.* New York, Holt, Rinehart and Winston, 1980, pp 51–52.

Jones IH, Horne DJdeL: Psychiatric disorders among Aborigines of the Australian western desert. *Soc Sci Med* 1973;7:219–228.

Kadrmas A, Winokur G, Growe R: Postpartum mania. *Br J Psychiatry* 1979; 135:551–554.

Kaij L, Nilsson A: Emotional and psychotic illness following childbirth, in Howells JG (ed): *Modern Perspectives in Psycho-obstetrics.* New York, Bruner/Mazel, 1972.

Katscher L: *Bilder aus dem Chinesischen Leben.* Leipzig, CF Winter, 1881.

Keeve JP, Schlesinger ER, Wight BW, Adams R: Fertility experience of juvenile girls: A community-wide ten-year study. *Am J Public Health* 1969;59:2185–2198.

Kiev A: Transcultural perspectives, in Hankoff LD, Einsidler B (eds): *Suicide: Theory and Clinical Aspects.* Littleton, Massachusetts, PSG Publishing, 1979, pp 215–224.

Kinsey AC, Pomeroy WB, Martin CE, Gebhard PH: *Sexual Behavior in the Human Female.* Philadelphia, WB Saunders, 1953.

Klaiber EL, Braverman DM, Vogel W, Kobayashi Y: Estrogen therapy for severe persistent depressions in women. *Arch Gen Psychiatry* 1979;36:550–554.
Kleiner GJ: Suicide in pregnancy. Special presentation at the Annual Meeting of the American Psychiatric Association. Chicago, May 16, 1979.
Kleiner, GJ, Hirsh J: Suicide in pregnancy. *Proceedings of the Fifth International Conference for Suicide Prevention* 1969, pp 170–171 (abstr).
Kloss M: Fatal gunshot wound of the foetus inflicted by the mother. *Aust NZ J Obstet Gynaecol* 1964;4:125–127.
Kreitman N, Smith P, Tan ES: Attempted suicide in social networks. *Br J Prev Soc Med* 1969;23:116–123.
Kretschmer E: *Körperbau und Character.* Berlin, Springer, 1951.
Kroger WS, Freed SC: *Psychosomatic Gynecology.* Philadelphia, WB Saunders, 1951.
Kumar R, Robson K: Neurotic disturbances during pregnancy and the puerperium, in Sandler M (ed): *Mental Illness in Pregnancy and the Puerperium.* New York, Oxford University Press, 1978.
LaFontaine J: Suicide among the Gisu, in Giddens A (ed): *The Sociology of Suicide. A Selection of Readings.* London, Frank Cass, 1971, pp 170–184.
Leifer M: Psychological changes accompanying pregnancy and motherhood. *Genet Psychol Monogr* 1977;95:55–96.
Lewis PJ: The effect of psychological drugs on the fetus, in Sandler M (ed): *Mental Illness in Pregnancy and the Puerperium.* New York, Oxford University Press, 1978, pp 99–111.
Lindberg BJ: Vad gör den abortsökande kvinnan, när psykiatern sagt nej? *Sven Läkartidn* 1948;45:1381 – cited by Ekblad, 1955, p 94.
Lindberg BJ: Psycho-infantilism. *Acta Psychiatr Scand* 1950;Suppl 61:1–126.
Lubin B, Gardener SH, Roth A: Mood and somatic symptoms during pregnancy. *Psychosom Med* 1975;37:136–146.
Lugo G, Cassady G, Palmisano P: Acute maternal arsenic intoxication with neonatal death. *Am J Dis Child* 1969;117:328–330.
Maas JW: Clinical and biochemical heterogeneity of depressive disorders. *Ann Intern Med* 1978;88:556–563.
MacKinnon IL, MacKinnon PCB, Thomson AD: Lethal hazards of the luteal phase of the menstrual cycle. *Br Med J* 1959;1:1015–1017.
Mandell AJ, Mandell MP: Suicide and the menstrual cycle. *JAMA* 1967;200:792–793.
Marce LV: *Traité de la Folie des Femmes Enceintes, des Nouvelles Accouchées et des Nourrices.* Paris, JB Sailliare et Fils, 1858.
Maris RW: *Social Forces in Urban Suicide.* Homewood, Illinois, Dorsey Press, 1969.
Masters WH, Johnson VE: *Human Sexual Response*. Boston, Little, Brown & Company, 1966.
Matějček Z, Dytrych Z, Schüller V: Children from unwanted pregnancies. *Acta Psychiatr Scand* 1978;57:67–90.
Maternal Deaths in the Commonwealth of Australia 1964–1975. *N.H. & M.R.C. Reports.* Canberra, Australian Government Publishing Service.
Maternal Mortality Committee: Minnesota maternal mortality study. *Minn Med* 1953;36:609–622.
McFarland J: *The Oxford Ibsen*, Vol VII. London, Oxford University Press, 1966, pp 167–352, 474–518.
McLure JN, Reich T, Wetzel RD: The menstrual cycle and suicide. *Br J Psychiatry* 1971;119:586–587.
McMurdo R: Pregnancy and suicide, in *Psychiatry for the Non-psychiatrist.* Sydney, Australia, Ciba-Geigy, undated, pp 92–95.

Morphew JA: Religion and attempted suicide. *Int J Soc Psychiatry* 1968;14:188–192.

Morris N: Attitude survey in pregnancy. *J Psychosom Res* 1968;12:83–84.

Nadelson CC: "Normal" and "special" aspects of pregnancy: A psychological approach, in Notman MT, Nadelson CC (eds): *The Woman Patient*, Vol 1. New York, Plenum Press, 1978.

Nashold RD: Attempted suicide by chemical agents. *Wis Med J* 1965;64:327–328.

Neale R: Attempted suicide in labour. *Br Med J* 1976;1:321–322.

Nelson FL, Farberow NL, MacKinnon DR: The certification of suicide in eleven western states: An inquiry into the validity of reported suicide rates. *Suicide Life Threat Behav* 1978;8:75–88.

New York City Department of Health, 1983: Statistics supplied by Frieda Nelson, Assistant Director, Bureau of Health Statistics and Analysis.

Nott PN, Franklin M, Armitage O, Gelder MG: Hormonal changes in mood in the puerperium. *Br J Psychiatry* 1976;128:379–383.

Oakley A: *Women Confined.* Oxford, Martin Robertson, 1980.

OSMA Committee on Maternal Health: Maternal deaths involving suicide. *Ohio State Med J* 1966;62:1294–1295.

OSMA Committee on Maternal and Neonatal Health: Maternal deaths involving suicide. *Ohio State Med J* 1976;72:711–712.

Otto U: Suicidal attempts made by pregnant women under 21 years. *Acta Paedopsychiatr (Basel)* 1965;32:276–288.

Otto U: Barns och ungdomars självmordshandlingar. – En barn och ungdomspsykiatrick studie Akademisk avhandling, Kristianstad, 1971.

Otto U: Suicidal acts by children and adolescents (a follow-up study). *Acta Psychiatr Scand* 1972;Suppl 233:1–123.

Otto U: Suicidal behavior in childhood and adolescence in suicide and attempted suicide. Skandia International Symposia. Nordiska bokhandelns förlag, Stockholm, 1972a, pp 189–204.

Otto U: Självmordshandlingar bland barn och ungdomar kröver aktivare uppföljning. *Nord Med* 1982;97:269–271.

Packard HL, Gampell R: Therpeutic abortion: A problem in law and medicine. *Stanford Law Rev* 1959;11:417.

Parker A: The meaning of attempted suicide to young parasuicides: A repertory grid study. *Br J Psychiatry* 1981;139:306–312.

Patel NS: A study of suicide. *Med Sci Law* 1974;14:134–135.

Paykel ES, Fletcher EJ, Rassaby ES: Life events and social support in puerperal depression. *Br J Psychiatry* 1980;136:339–346.

Pitt B: Atypical depression following childbirth. *Br J Psychiatry* 1968;114:1325–1335.

Planned Parenthood Federation of America: *Abortion in the United States.* Calderone MS (ed): New York, Hoeber-Harper, 1958, p 140.

Ploss H, Bartels H: *Das Weib in der Natur-und Volkerkunde,* Vol 2. Leipzig, Grieben, 1905, pp 712–768.

Pokorny AD: The Scandinavian suicide phenomenon – myth or reality? *Suicide Life Threat Behav* 1973;3:11–19.

Potondi A: Selbstmord und schwangerschaft. *Dtsche Z Gerichtl Med* 1965; 56:172–176.

Price J, Karim I: Suicide in Fiji: A two-year survey. *Acta Psychiatr Scand* 1975; 52:153–159.

Pritchard JA, MacDonald PC: *Williams Obstetrics,* 15th ed. New York, Appleton-Century-Crofts, 1976.

Pritchard JA, MacDonald PC: *Williams Obstetrics,* 16th ed. New York, Appleton-Century-Crofts, 1980.

Pugh TF, Jerath BK, Schmidt WM, Reed RB: Rates of mental disease related to childbearing. *N Engl J Med* 1963;268:1224–1228.

Reich T, Winokur G: Postpartum psychosis in patients with manic-depressive disease. *J Nerv Ment Dis* 1970;151:60–68.

Report on Confidential Enquiries into Maternal Deaths in England and Wales 1952–1954: *Ministry of Health Reports on Public Health and Medical Subjects No. 97.* London, Her Majesty's Stationery Office, 1957.

Report on Confidential Enquiries into Maternal Deaths in England and Wales 1955–1957: *Ministry of Health Reports on Public Health and Medical Subjects No. 103.* London, Her Majesty's Stationery Office, 1960.

Report on Confidential Enquiries into Maternal Deaths in England and Wales 1958–1960: *Ministry of Health Reports on Public Health and Medical Subjects No. 108.* London, Her Majesty's Stationery Office, 1963.

Report on Confidential Enquiries into Maternal Deaths in England and Wales 1961–1963: *Ministry of Health Reports on Public Health and Medical Subjects No. 115.* London, Her Majesty's Stationery Office, 1966.

Report on Confidential Enquiries into Maternal Deaths in England and Wales 1964–1966: *Department of Health and Social Security Reports on Public Health and Medical Subjects No. 119.* London, Her Majesty's Stationery Office, 1969.

Report on Confidential Enquiries into Maternal Deaths in England and Wales 1967–1969: *Department of Health and Social Security Reports on Health and Social Subjects No. 1.* London, Her Majesty's Stationery Office, 1972.

Report on Confidential Enquiries into Maternal Deaths in England and Wales 1970–1972: *Department of Health and Social Security Reports on Health and Social Subjects No. 11.* London, Her Majesty's Stationery Office, 1975.

Report on Confidential Enquiries into Maternal Deaths in England and Wales 1973–1975: *Department of Health and Social Security Reports on Health and Social Subjects No. 14.* London, Her Majesty's Stationery Office, 1979.

Resnik HLP, Wittlin BJ: Abortion and suicidal behaviors: Observations on the concept of "endangering the mental health of the mother." *Ment Hygiene* 1971; 55:10–20.

Ribeiro AL: Menstruation and crime. *Br Med J* 1962;1:640.

Richards R, Brooks SEH: Ferrous sulphate poisoning in pregnancy (with afibrinogenaemia as a complication). *West Indian Med J* 1966;15:134–140.

Rodenbury M: Child murder by depressed parents. *Can Psychiatr Assoc J* 1971; 16:41–48.

Rosen H: Psychiatric implications of abortion: A case study in social hypocrisy. *West Reserve Law Rev* 1965;17:445.

Rosenberg A, Silver E: Suicide, psychiatrists and therapeutic abortion. *Calif Med* 1965;102:407–411.

Rubenstein R, Moses R, Lidz T: On attempted suicide. *AMA Arch Neurol Psychiatr* 1958;79:103–112.

Sainsbury P: Suicide: Opinion and facts. *Proc R Soc Med* 1973;66:579–587.

Sainsbury P, Jenkins JS: The accuracy of officially reported suicide statistics for purposes of epidemiological research. *J Epidemiol Community Health* 1982; 36:43–48.

Saks BR: What can you do for the depressed patient? *Contemp Ob/Gyn* 1981; 18:71–77.

Saks BR, Frank J, Naftolin F, Lowe TL, Berman W, Cohen DJ: Current psychoneuroendocrine research on postpartum depression (in press).

Sandler M: *Mental Illness in Pregnancy and the Puerperium.* New York, Oxford University Press, 1978.

Sarrel PM, Davis CD: The young unwed primipara. A study of 100 cases with 5 year follow-up. *Am J Obstet Gynecol* 1966;95:722–725.

Sarrel PM, Klerman LV: The young unwed mother—obstetric results of a program of comprehensive care. *Am J Obstet Gynecol* 1969;105:575–578.

Schleisinger RH, Davis CD, Milliken SO: Outpatient care—the influence of interrelated needs. *Am J Public Health* 1962;52:1844–1852.

Schmidt EH, O'Neal P, Robins E: Evaluation of suicide attempts as guide to therapy. Clinical and follow-up study of 109 patients. *JAMA* 1954;155:549–557.

Schou M, Amdisen A: Lithium and pregnancy III. Lithium ingestion by children breastfed by women on lithium. *Br Med J* 1973;2:138.

Sclare AB, Hamilton CM: Attempted suicide in Glasgow. *Br J Psychiatry* 1963; 109:609–615.

Seager CP, Flood RA: Suicide in Bristol. *Br J Psychiatry* 1965;111:919–932.

Seiden RH: *Suicide Among Youth: A Supplement to the Bulletin of Suicidology.* National Clearinghouse for Mental Health Information, National Institute of Mental Health, Rockville, Maryland, 1969.

Shader RI, DiMascio A: *Psychotropic Drug Side Effects.* Baltimore, Williams & Wilkins, 1970.

Shainess N: Psychological problems associated with motherhood, in Arieti S (ed): *American Handbook of Psychiatry,* Vol 3. New York, Basic Books, 1966, pp 47–65.

Shakespeare W: *The Plays and Poems of William Shakespeare, with the Corrections and Illustrations of Various Commentators,* by the late Edmond Malone, Vol 20. London, C. Baldwin, 1821, pp 93–214.

Shakespeare W: *The Tragedy of Hamlet, Prince of Denmark (1604–1605).* Baltimore, Maryland, Penguin Books, 1957, pp 73, 132–133.

Shereshefsky PM, Yarrow LJ: *Psychological Aspects of a First Pregnancy and Early Postnatal Adaptation.* New York, Raven Press, 1973.

Shneidman ES, Farberow NL: Clues to suicide. *Public Health Rep* 1956;71:109–114.

Shneidman ES, Farberow NL: Statistical comparisons between attempted and committed suicides, in Farberow NL, Shneidman ES (eds): *The Cry for Help.* New York, McGraw-Hill, 1961.

Sichel P: *Modigliani.* New York, EP Dutton, 1967, pp 465–522.

Siegel LJ, Friedman JH: The threat of suicide. *Dis Nerv Syst* 1955;16:37–46.

Silverblatt H, Goodwin J: The denial of pregnancy. Presented at the 6th World Congress of the International College of Psychosomatic Medicine. Montreal, September 13–18, 1981.

Silving H: Suicide and law, in Shneidman ES, Farberow NL (eds): *Clues to Suicide.* New York, McGraw-Hill, 1957, pp 79–95.

Sim M: Abortion and the psychiatrist. *Br Med J* 1963;2:145–148.

Sim M: Psychiatric disorders of pregnancy. *J Psychosom Res* 1968;12:95–100.

Slochower H: Suicides in literature; their ego function. *Am Imago* 1975;32:389–416.

Snyder BJ: A note on the importance of cultural factors in suicide studies. *Suicide Life Threat Behav* 1977;7:230–235.

Sobel DE: Fetal damage due to ECT, insulin coma, chlorpromazine or reserpine. *Arch Gen Psychiatry* 1960;2:606–611.

Socialstyrelsen: Medicinalväsendets författningssamling. MF 1974:76.

SOU 1953/29—Statans Offentliga Utredningar 1953, No. 29, Abortfrågan, Betänkande avgivet av 1950 års abortutredning. Stockholm, 1953.

SOU 1964/40—Statens offentliga utredningar: Mentalsjukvårdslag. Betänkande avgivet av sinnessjuklagstiftningskommitten. Stockholm, 1964.

SOU 1971/58—Statens offentliga utredningar: Rätten till abort. 1965 års abortkommitte, Stockholm, 1971.

Spring H: *My Son, My Son.* New York, Viking, 1938, pp 461–548.

Sriwatanakul K, Weis O: Using antipsychotic drugs during pregnancy. *Drug Ther* 1982;12:97–99.

Stengel E: Recent research into suicide and attempted suicide. *Am J Psychiatry* 1962;118:725–727.

Stengel E, Cook NG: *Attempted Suicide: Its Social Significance and Effects.* London, Institute of Psychiatry, 1958.

Stern ES: The Medea complex: Mother's homicidal wishes to her children. *J Ment Sci* 1978;94:321–331.

Suicide risk in teenage pregnancy (editorial). *Br Med J* 1971;2:602.

Suicide statistics: The problem of comparability. *WHO Chronicle* 1975;29:188–193.

Sveriges officiella statistik: Socialstyrelsen. Allmän hälso-och sjukvård, 1978.

Sveriges officiella statistik: Statistisk årsbok, 1981, S 292–295.

Sweeney D, Maas JW: Specificity of depressive diseases. *Annu Rev Med* 1978; 29:219–229.

Szabo KT, Brent RL: Species differences in experimental teratogenesis by tranquilizing agents. *Lancet* 1974;1:565.

Szasz TS: The ethics of birth control. *The Humanist* 1960;20:322.

Takki S, Pollanen P, Lebtonen T: Criminal abortion by gunshot. A case report. *Ann Chir Gynaecol Fenn* 1969;58:122–123.

Tangum SD, Davenport YB, Webster MJ: Postpartum mania in bipolar manic depressive patients withdrawn from lithium carbonate. *J Nerv Ment Dis* 1979; 167:572–574.

Taylor DJE, Hart FD, Burley D: Suicide in South London. An analysis of the admissions for attempted suicide in one medical unit of a general hospital. *Practitioner* 1964;192:251–256.

Taylor SE, Langer EJ: Pregnancy: Social stigma? *Sex Roles J Res* 1977;3:27–36.

Thomas CL, Gordon JE: Psychosis after childbirth: Ecological aspects of a single impact stress. *Am J Med Sci* 1959;238:363–388.

Thonet C: Frustrated suicide during pregnancy. *Rev Chil Obstet Ginecol* 1967; 32:166–170.

Thurston G: Forensic medicine and toxicology. Reference to the coroner. *Br Med J* 1967;2:361–362.

Tishler CL: Adolescent suicide attempts following elective abortion: A special case of anniversary reaction. *Pediatrics* 1981;68:670–671.

Treadway CR, Kane FJ Jr, Jarrahi-Zadeh A, Linton MA: A psychoendocrine study of pregnancy and the puerperium. *Am J Psychiatry* 1969;125:1380–1385.

Turneer MF, Izzi MH: The COPE story: A service to pregnant and postpartum women, in Notman MT, Nadelson CC (eds): *The Woman Patient,* Vol 1. New York, Plenum Press, 1978, pp 107–136.

Tylden E: Psychiatric disorders including drug therapy and addiction. *Clin Obstet Gynaecol* 1977;4(2):435–439.

U.S. Vital Statistics, 1982: *Vital Statistics of the United States—1978,* Vol 1 (Natality). U.S. Department of Health and Human Services. Public Health Services. Washington, US Govt Printing Office, 1982, pp 1–72.

Veevers JE: Parenthood and suicide: An examination of a neglected variable. *Soc Sci Med* 1973;7:135–144.

Veith I: Reflections on the medical history of suicide. *Mod Med* 1969;38:116–121.

Von Sury K: *Muench Med Wochenschr* 1908;55:1534–1536.

Waddell WJ, Marlow L: Transfer of drugs across the placenta. *Pharmacol Ther* 1981;14:375–390.

Weissman MM, Klerman GL: Sex differences and the epidemiology of depression. *Arch Gen Psychiatry* 1977;34:98–111.

Wen CP: Secular suicidal trend in postwar Japan and Taiwan. An examination of hypotheses. *Int J Soc Psychiatry* 1974;20:8–17.

Wenner NK, Cohen MB, Weigert EV, Kvarnes RG, Ohaneson EM, Fearing JM: Emotional problems in pregnancy. *Psychiatry* 1969;32:389–410.

When Children Bear Children: *New York Times,* August 1, 1983 (editorial).

Whitlock FA, Edwards JE: Pregnancy and attempted suicide. *Compr Psychiatry* 1968;9:1–12.

Whitlock FA: Depression and suicide, in Burrows G (ed): *Handbook of Studies of Depression.* Amsterdam, Elsevier, 1977, pp 379–403.

Wilson AR: An investigation into the psychological aspects of pregnancy and the puerperium using the techniques of group analysis. *J Psychosom Res* 1968; 12:73–82.

Wintour EM, Coghlan JP, Oddie CJ, Scoggins BA, Walters WAW: A sequential study of adrenocorticosteroid level in human pregnancy. *Clin Exp Pharmacol Physiol* 1978;5:399–403.

Woodis GM, Robinson GA: Attempted suicide during the course of labour. *Med Leg J* 1960;28:209–211.

World Health Organization: *Suicide and Attempted Suicide* (Public Health Papers No. 58). Geneva, World Health Organization, 1974, pp 1–127.

Wren CS: Old nemesis haunts China on birth plan. *New York Times,* August 1, 1982, p 9.

Yalon ID, Lunde PT, Moos RH, Hamburg DA: Postpartum blues syndrome. *Arch Gen Psychiatry* 1968;18:16–27.

Yarrow HC: A further contribution to the study of the mortuary customs of the North American Indians, in Powell JW: *First Annual Report of the Bureau of Ethnology to the Secretary of the Smithsonian Institute, 1879–1880.* Washington, 1881.

Youngs DD, Lucas MJ: Postpartum depression: Hormonal versus alternate perspectives, in Youngs DD, Ehrhardt AA (eds): *Psychosomatic Obstetrics and Gynecology.* New York, Appleton-Century-Crofts, 1980.

INDEX

An asterisk (*) after a page number denotes data to be found in a table or figure.